PALEO MADE EASY:

GETTING YOUR FAMILY STARTED WITH THE OPTIMAL HEALTHY LIFESTYLE

Sylvie McCracken of HollywoodHomestead.com

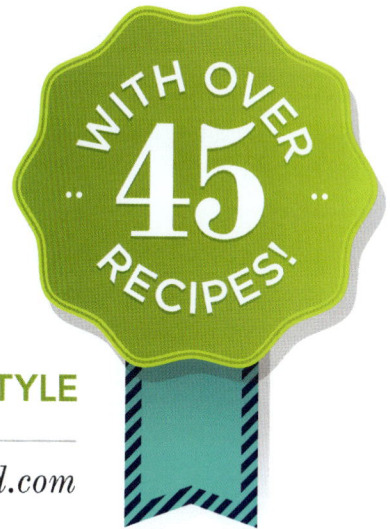

WITH OVER **45** RECIPES!

Paleo Made Easy: Getting your Family Started with the Optimal Healthy Lifestyle—with over 45 recipes!

Sylvie McCracken of HollywoodHomestead.com
Copyright 2013 Sylvie McCracken

ISBN: 978-0-9861460-0-8

Disclaimer and Copyright Information

HH

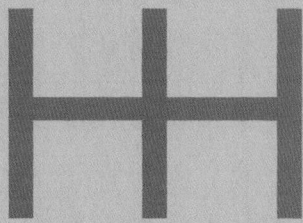

HOLLYWOOD
HOMESTEAD

CONTENTS

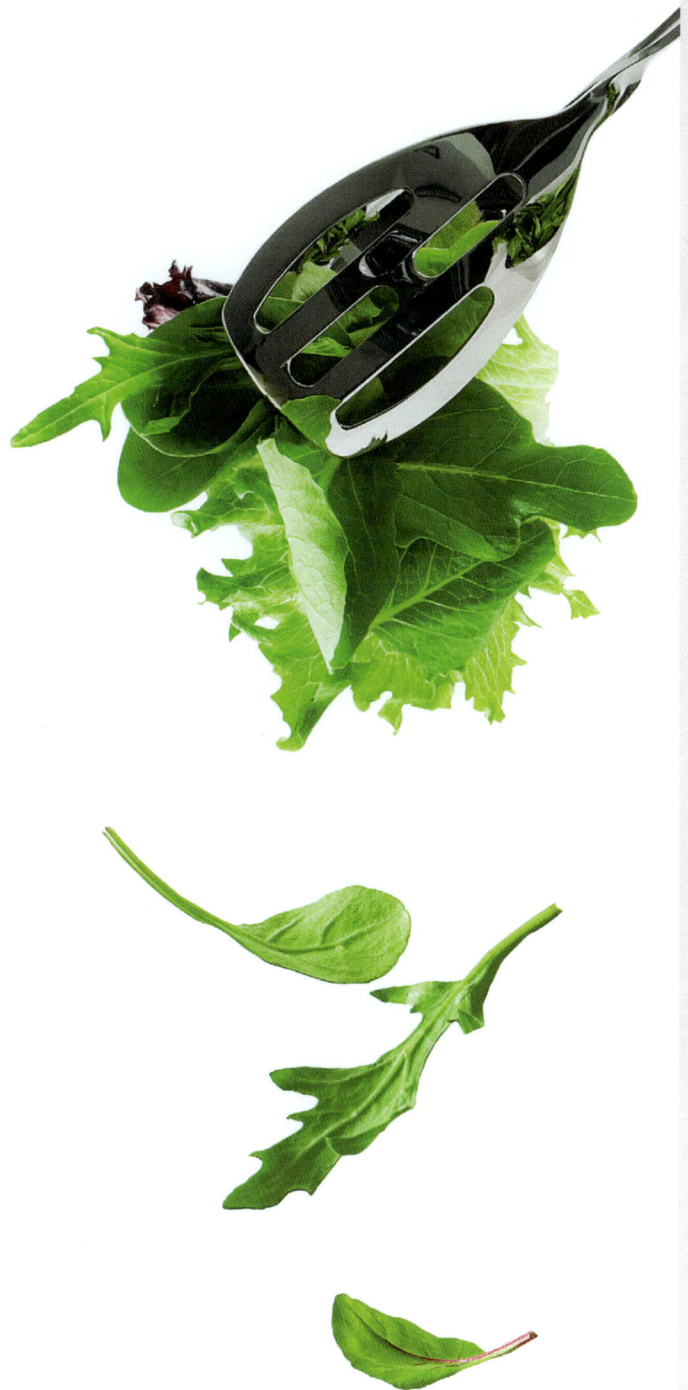

ABOUT THE AUTHOR

Sylvie was raised in Argentina but currently lives in Los Angeles where she juggles a fast-paced career as an Executive Assistant to an Oscar-winning actor while managing to get the real food word out to celebrities and civilians alike.

Sylvie and Eric each lost over 60 lbs in the first year of adopting a paleo diet. You can read their paleo success stories on pages 7–9.

On weekends, Sylvie, Eric and their three kids can be found in the kitchen, the garden, the beach or hiking, and sometimes a combo of all of the above.

You can find out more about their lifestyle at the blog www.hollywoodhomestead.com and follow them on Facebook, Twitter, Pinterest, and Instagram.

Sign up for our newsletter at: http://www.hollywoodhomestead.com/sign-up

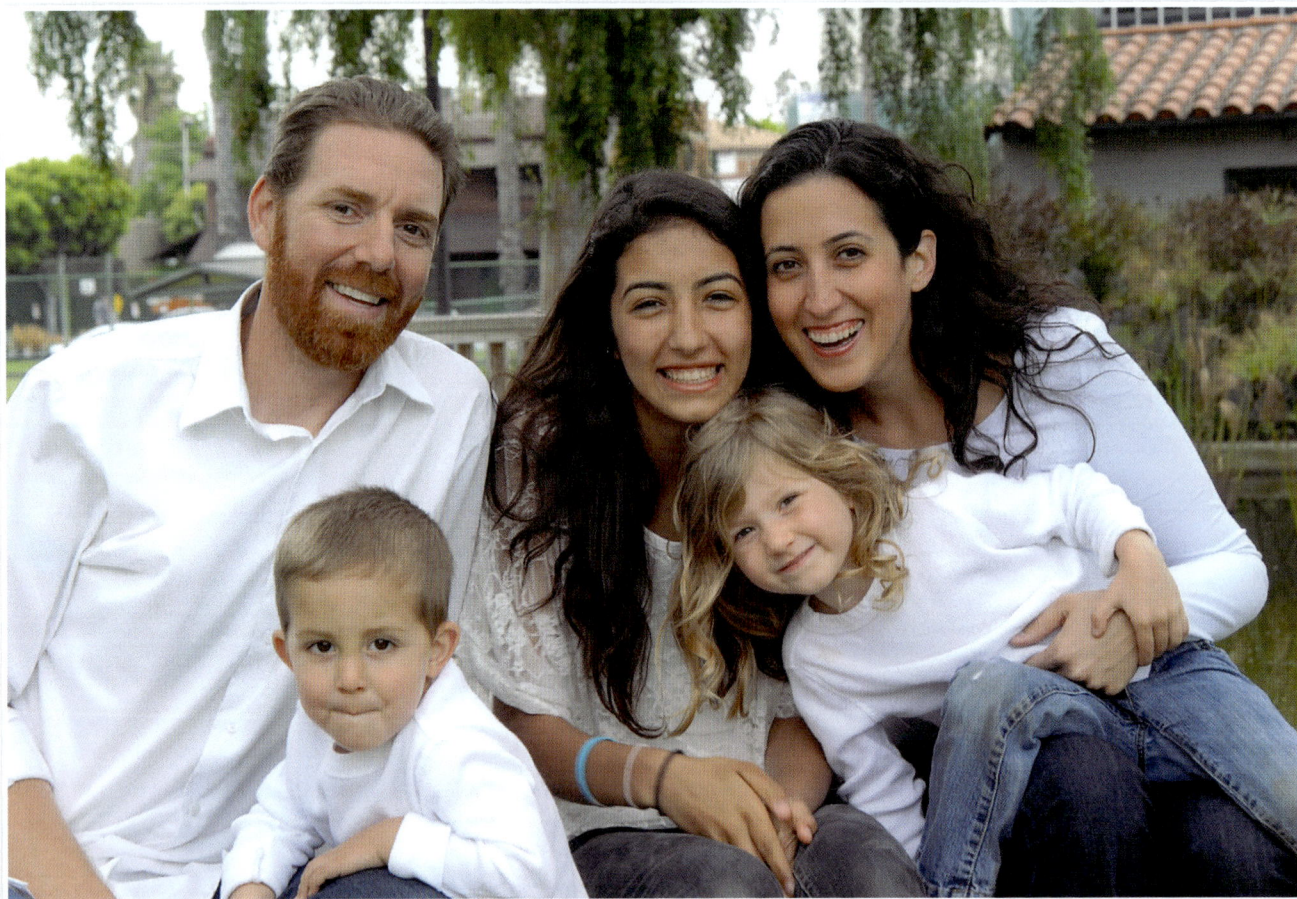

Photo by Selma Al-Faqih

Paleo Made Easy: Getting your Family Started with the Optimal Healthy Lifestyle—with over 45 recipes!

PALEO SUCCESS STORIES

SYLVIE'S PALEO JOURNEY

I've lost 65 lbs with paleo but, really, that's just the cherry on top.

I didn't get into the paleo lifestyle to lose weight. I'd sort of given up on the weight-loss front. After hitting age 30 and having had 3 kids, I assumed there's only so much one can do.

I was not an overweight kid but I was definitely a health disaster. I was a lacto-ovo vegetarian for most of my childhood and consumed mostly soy and wheat with a few lentils thrown in for good measure. By age 15 my list of diagnoses was impressive and the medications were starting to pile up:

- Polycystic ovarian syndrome

- Chronic Amenhorrea = Rx: birth control

- Hypothyroid = Rx: Synthroid

- Tonsillitis and strep throat at least yearly=Rx: many rounds of Amoxicillin, later large doses of penicillin and finally tonsillectomy

- Chronic allergic rhinitis = Rx: cortisone nasal spray and decongestants (which I became addicted to) and eventually nasal polyps which were surgically removed during my teen years in addition to cryosurgery on my adenoids. Fun times.

- Allergic to just about everything = Rx: allergy shots every 4 days starting as a pre-teen that I would self administer after school

- Epstein-Barr virus (aka "mono") multiple times = Rx: rest, hope and prayer (ha!)

- All of this was in addition to a heart condition I was born with called supraventricular tachycardia for which I was on beta blockers and other random things that never worked until I had my heart catheter ablation when I was 21.

Comprehensive diagnosis: HOT MESS

My medical file was a FAT one (pun intended)! Seriously, when my mom handed it off to me a few years ago, even I was shocked.

My experiment with paleo came out of desperation since my thyroid symptoms (fatigue being the most crippling one) were persistent and severe despite my lab work being "normal". The first 30 days of the transition to paleo were **not** easy. My body was not used to so much animal protein and fat, and I was dealing with mad cravings for sugar and wheat. Finding the time, energy and money to do more shopping, cooking and dishes while juggling the usual madness of life definitely took some effort for both me and my husband Eric.

We made mistakes.

We got frustrated.

But, we stuck with it.

I lost 65 lbs with paleo. The craziest part was that I wasn't focusing on weight loss at all.

I realize there's many ways to lose weight. I've tried many of them myself: calorie counting, low fat, more exercise, low carb, slim fast, cortisol regulating supplements, among others. Some of them were seemingly successful, but I'd eventually gain the few pounds I lost right back.

You see, being overweight or underweight is often not the problem. It is a symptom of a problem. When you're body finds health, it will most likely self-adjust on the weight front quite a bit.

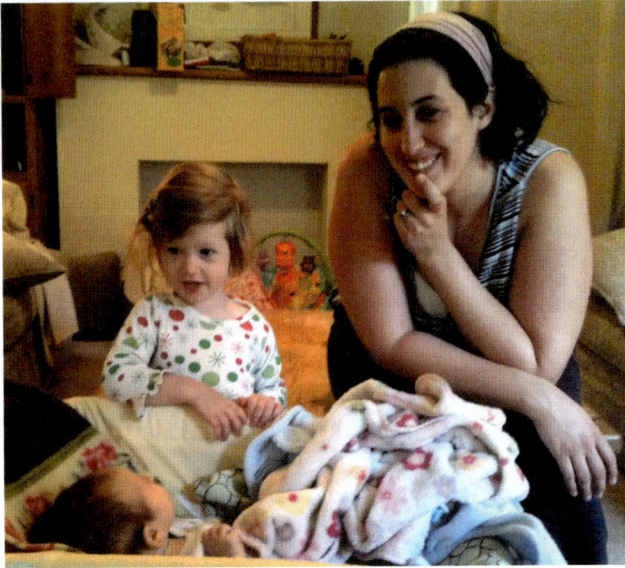

The improvements I found with paleo were well beyond weight loss:

- My cycle is like clockwork now. I'd asked countless MDs about this and only received shoulder shrugs and pre-scriptions for birth control.

- My blood sugar (and hence mood) is finally regulated.

- The bags under my eyes which I thought were hereditary and obsessively covered with makeup are gone (unless those little kids keep me up at night) :)

- My nails don't break as easily. My teeth are not translu-cent and I have not had a cavity since going paleo. This is someone that had a cavity at EVERY SINGLE dental visit- and no, my diet was not nothing but pop tarts.

The reason that I attained these benefits from paleo was because **I was malnourished.**

I was fat yet malnourished. It sounds paradoxical, but it's true.

Food really is medicine.

In the last few months I've started working with a natu-ropath to help me continue to achieve optimal health. I will always be a work in progress and have many years of damage to unravel. After three decades of consuming large amounts of soy, wheat and very little animal protein and fat, my body just can't handle everything as it was meant to on its own. This process is sometimes discouraging but, most of the time, it's fascinating and uplifting.

I've only just begun my journey of finding health and I'm honored you're giving me the opportunity to help you do the same!

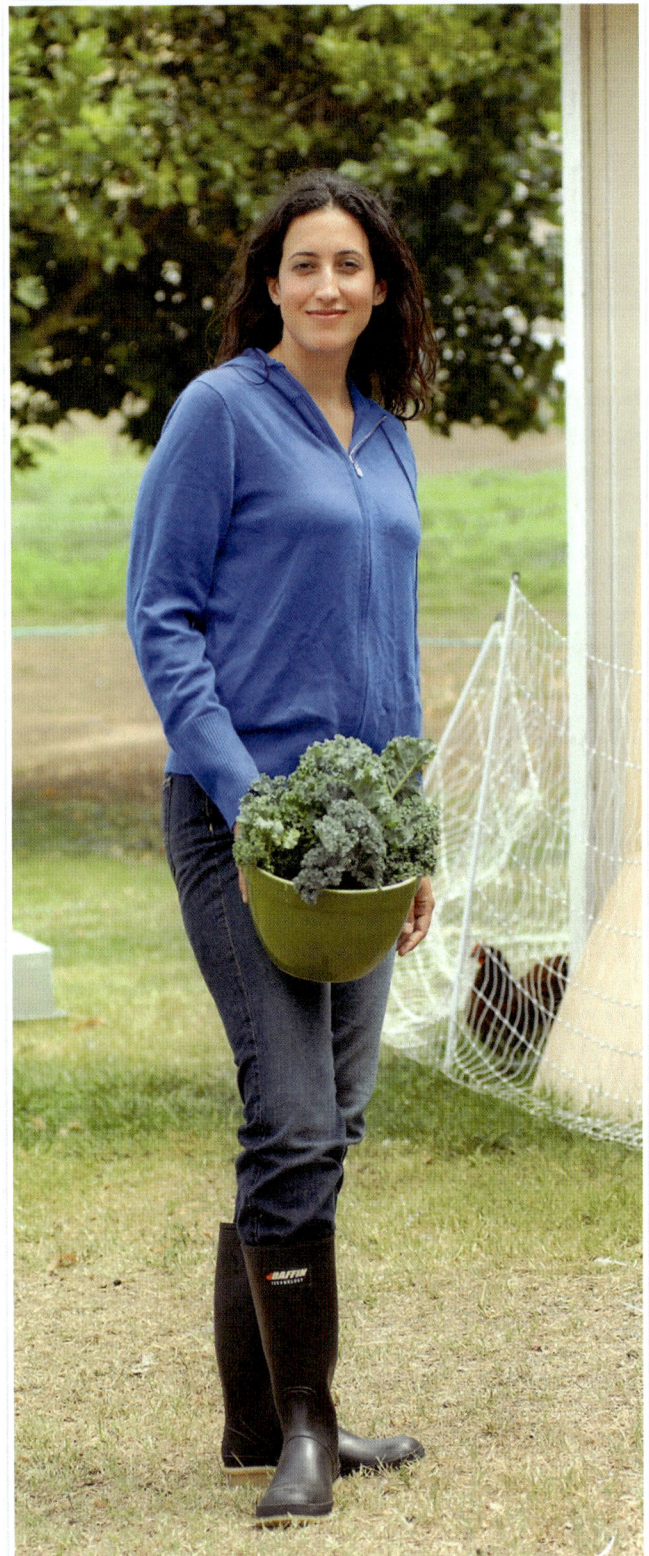

Photo by Selma Al-Faqih

Paleo Made Easy: Getting your Family Started with the Optimal Healthy Lifestyle—with over 45 recipes!

ERIC'S PALEO JOURNEY

What is the Paleo question?

I didn't know the Paleo question when I started this journey with Sylvie. Here is what I did know: I felt slow and sluggish. I got winded easily. My joints hurt. The vision in my right eye was getting worse. I was on a hunger and blood sugar roller coaster—I went from too full to starving every few hours. It was tough to lose weight. My ideal weight in my mind was continuing to rise... 185... 195... I'll be happy under 200... 205 isn't that bad... everyone aspires to be at the weight they were when they got married, right? 205 is great! I feel fine...

I was lying to myself. I was *NOT* feeling fine.

I think the Paleo question is WHY? Why am I sluggish? Why do my joints hurt? Why is my vision getting worse? Why did I feel awful after eating and then starving a few hours later?

The standard answers to these questions are easy: You're getting older. You're overweight.

Standard "solutions" to these answers didn't work for me: Reduce portion size. Exercise. Been there, done that. I'd lose weight and gain it right back again.

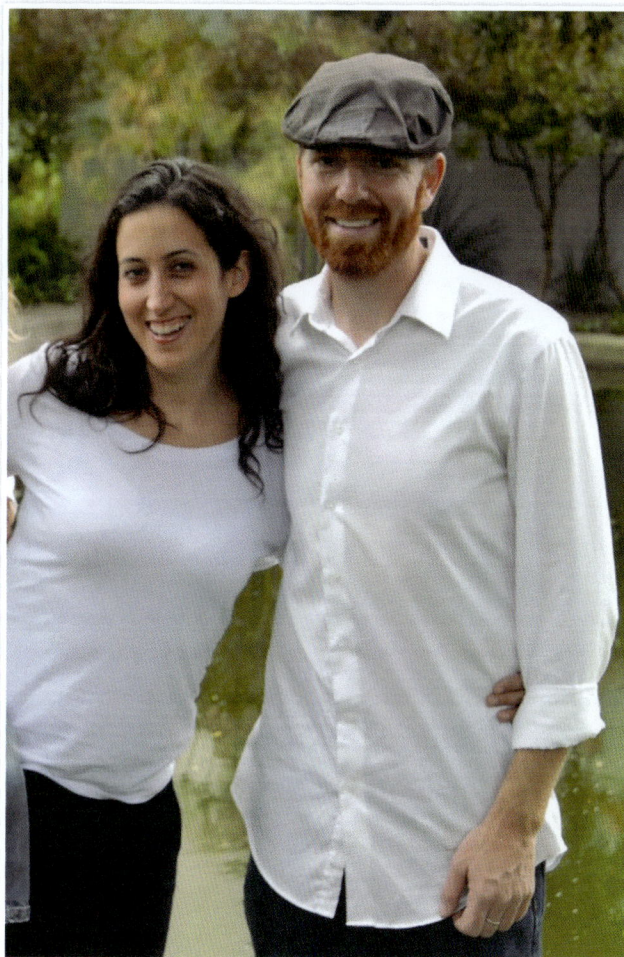

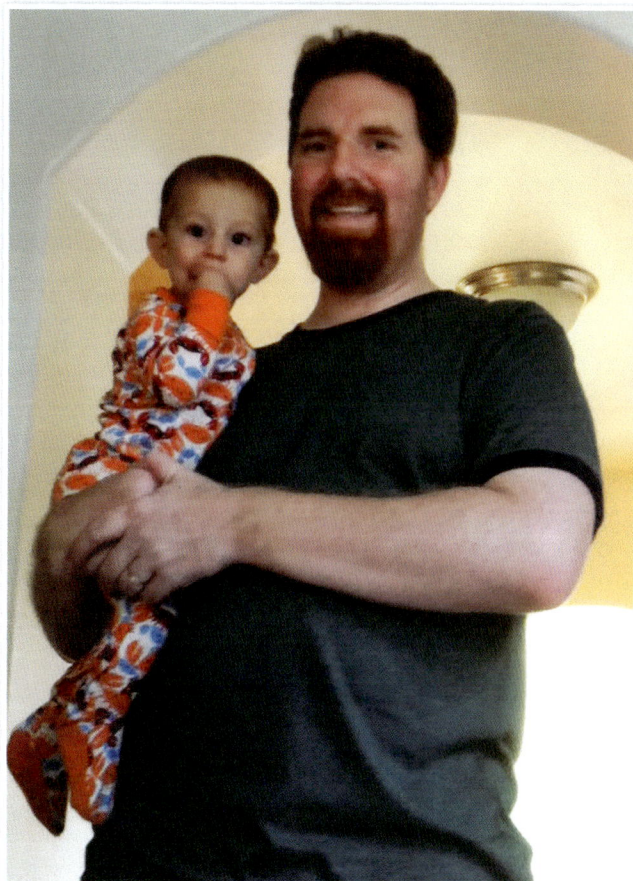

I wanted *off* the roller coaster.

When I came home after 7 months of being in Abu Dhabi without my wife and children, I weighed 235 pounds. Sylvie and I knew that something had to change.

That is when we stumbled upon paleo. Sylvie started right away, but I was skeptical. But then Sylvie started to feel better so I decided to give it a try.

That was almost a year ago. I am now 170 pounds. The vision in my right eye is fine. My joints don't hurt. I have energy again. I feel light on my feet. The best part? I eat as much as I want and I don't think about calories. *I can't gain weight!* I got off the roller coaster and life is good. I see a field and I know I can sprint to the other side with my kids and actually beat them there. I have a 14 year old, so that's not easy!

The great thing about the paleo answer is that it has us questioning *everything*. The bottom line is that only *we* have our best interests at heart. If we want to succeed in health, in finance, in life, *we* have to find the right answers for *us*.

The best way to start is to ask the right questions.

INTRODUCTION

If you had told me before I started this paleo journey I'd be writing an ebook and teaching online classes about nutrition and health that would have cracked.me.up. I had no idea what I was doing. I didn't know where to start. I thought cayenne pepper and lemon would be the answer to all my problems.

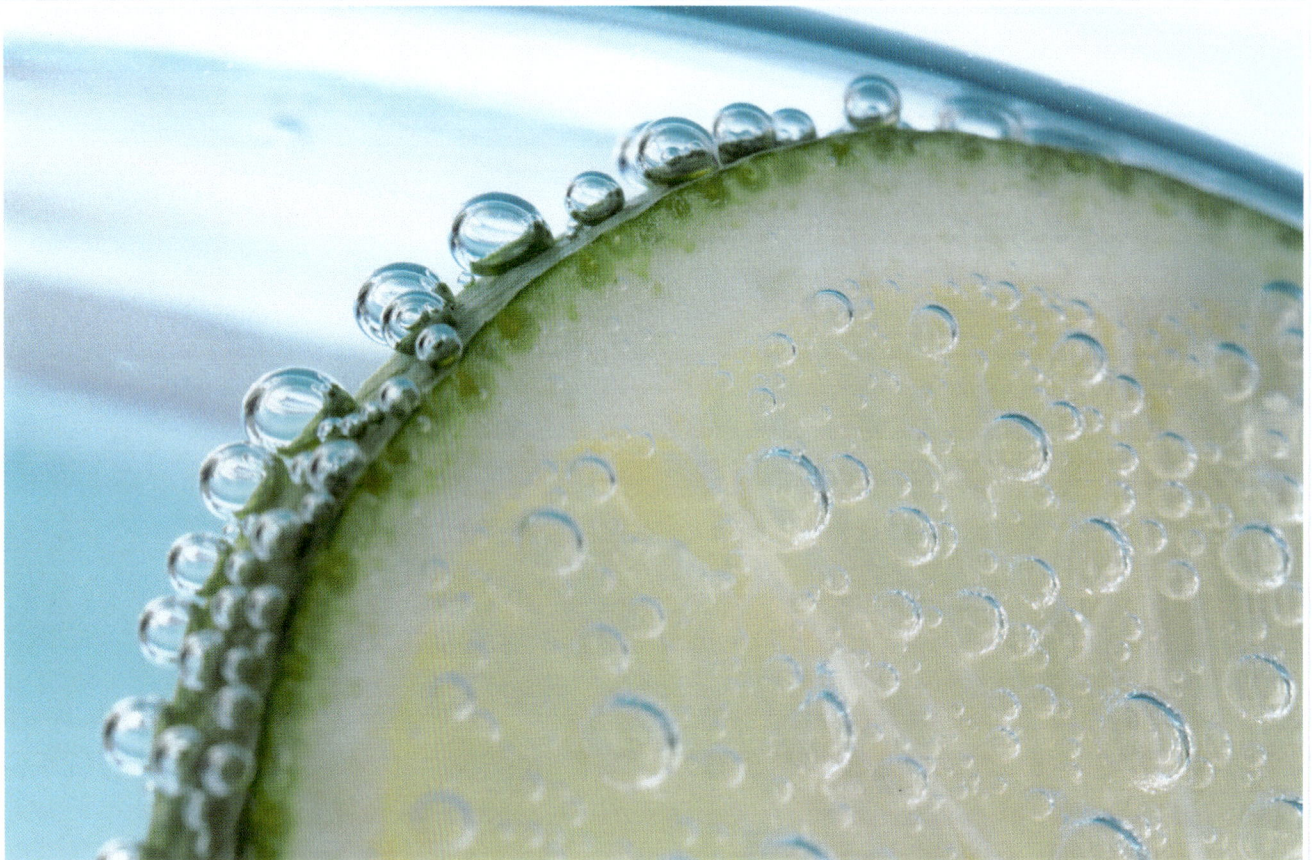

Over the last couple of years I have studied, experimented, listened, written, argued, discussed and absorbed as much information on nutrition and lifestyle as possible. I've swapped vacations for conferences and tv shows for seminars.

I eat, sleep and breathe paleo nutrition and lifestyle. I started my website and facebook page because I just couldn't keep all of this to myself.

Every time my before and after photos are picked up in the interwebs I have an influx of people coming to me saying *"you look great! I want to do this! How do I start?"*.

It became apparent that tell you to *just start doing it* is not comprehensive enough. I've heard your requests and I have put everything in one place for you so that you can do just that: **START!**

My hope is that this book will answer any question or concern that you have and help you bust any excuse that may be holding you back from achieving the life you deserve.

My goal was to write the guide I wish I had been led to when my doctor told me I needed to make changes.

As always, if you have additional questions please hop over to the Facebook page and let's chat!

CHAPTER 1

WHAT IS PALEO?

Paleo is short for paleolithic as in... a hell of a long time ago.

You may have heard the paleo diet requires you to eat like our cavemen ancestors did and toss your laptop out the window while you're at it. I'm not a big fan of dogma. It usually only leads to arguing with strangers online, when you're not looking at pictures of sloths and ain't nobody got time for that!

So, why do I choose paleo to describe my diet? Because paleo is the closest way to describe the way my family and I try to eat and live most of the time.

What do you eat and not eat on a paleo diet?

EAT	DON'T EAT
Meat of all kinds (preferably pastured)—bonus points for organ meat!	Grains (especially gluten containing grains like wheat, rye and barley)
Fish (preferably wild caught)	Legumes (including peanuts)
Eggs (preferably pastured)	Dairy (although many include raw grass-fed full fat dairy if tolerated well)
Vegetables (preferably local, seasonal and organic)	Processed foods
Fat, yes even saturated fat (from pastured animals, avocados, coconut, etc)	Refined sugar
Fermented foods and beverages	Alcohol
Fruit (preferably local, seasonal and organic)	
Nuts and seeds (if you tolerate them well)	

Paleo Made Easy: Getting your Family Started with the Optimal Healthy Lifestyle—with over 45 recipes!

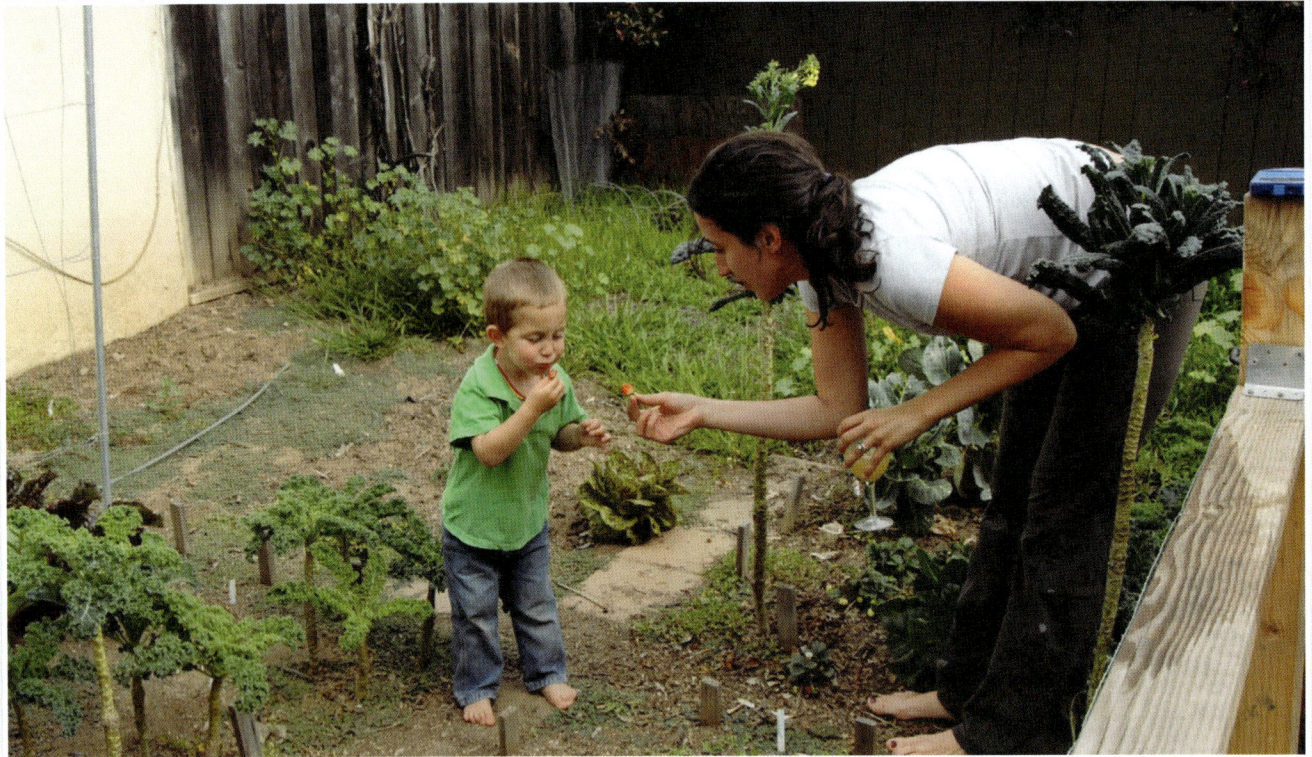

Other similar Real Food approaches are Primal (which includes raw grass-fed dairy), and Weston A. Price (which includes raw, grass-fed dairy as well as soaked, sprouted and fermented grains). All of these approaches would fall under the category of "ancestral" or traditional.

So back to what paleo is... to me at least.

Paleo is about eating *real* food, NUTRIENT DENSE food, food our ancestors would have recognized, food that is grown in the ground or roams the earth, and food that is minimally processed and doesn't come packaged in a box or bag with a shelf life of practically forever.

Paleo is crowding out less nutritious, pro-inflammatory foods like grains. It is an anti-inflammatory diet, hence the incredible results in people with autoimmune and other diseases.

Does that mean that my family roams around the backyard grabbing handfuls of produce and inserting it into our mouths without so much as a rinse? Well, sometimes...

But most of the time we just do our best to plan, shop and prepare meat and vegetables at each meal and have some fruit and nuts available as well, especially for the growing kids. Does it mean we never buy anything in a package or off a shelf? Of course not! We love our occasional paleo treats and the 80/20 rule is what makes paleo sustainable for us in the long term.

WHY ADOPT A PALEO DIET?

I stumbled upon paleo sort of by accident, when my doctor suspected for several months that I had an autoimmune disease. That was enough to get my attention and start me Googling like mad to see what I could do to reverse it.

One of the many lab tests I had done was a leaky gut test that confirmed that my intestinal barrier was indeed very permeable. Leaky gut is exactly what it sounds like: the intestine is permeable and allows undigested particles of food, bacteria and even bits of your intestinal lining into your bloodstream. In summary: *no bueno!* The body makes antibodies for these foreign invaders (bits of food and whatnot have no business in the bloodstream) and later on this can lead to an autoimmune attack in which is your body attacking its own tissues, which it does not recognize. Yikes!

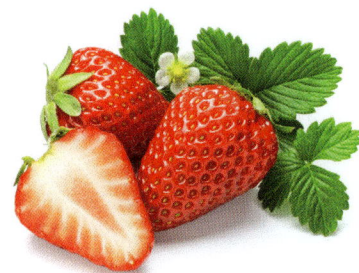

Paleo Made Easy: Getting your Family Started with the Optimal Healthy Lifestyle—with over 45 recipes!

WHY CHOOSE PALEO OVER WESTON A. PRICE OR TRADITIONAL FOODS DIETS

Let's face it, if you have leaky gut after years of eating less-than-optimal foods and your body is in a constant state of inflammation, then it is time to pay the piper. That means getting rid of every food that is not optimal in gut healing and including plenty of gut healing foods like grass-fed gelatin and bone broth.

For many of us, grains and legumes are difficult to digest even when properly prepared according to Weston A. Price principles and the lecithin, phytic acid and anti nutrients in grains and legumes can further irritate an already sensitive gut.

ISN'T PALEO JUST ANOTHER LOW CARB DIET?

One common misconception of the paleo diet is that it is low carb. It is definitely much lower in carbs than the Standard American Diet and can also be lower carb than traditional foods diets that include grains and legumes. However, a much more accurate description of a paleo diet is *low crap diet*. In other words, no processed foods.

How many carbs you choose to include in paleo is up to you and your goals. I personally don't do well when I eat too few carbs, so I make sure to include potatoes, sweet potatoes, cauliflower or other carbohydrate-rich vegetables at every meal. Other people thrive on a lower carb and even a ketogenic approach.

IS A PALEO DIET SAFE FOR CHILDREN?

Not only is it safe for children, it is often life changing! I have 3 kids and have seen astounding changes in all of them since we adopted a paleo diet. My teen's acne has significantly improved and my preschoolers are much better in control of their bodies and emotions. I have no doubt my 4 year old would have been prescribed medication eventually if it weren't for the dietary shifts.

HOW DO I KNOW IF PALEO IS RIGHT FOR ME?

The paleo diet has worked wonders for me and my family. But how do you know if it will work for you? The best way to know is to simply try it. Ideally, you would try it for 30 days so you can really experience the benefits and be able to compare how you feel on and off grains. But, if that sounds overwhelming, perhaps you can just give it a shot for 1 week and reevaluate then. What's the worst that can happen? You'll likely lose a few pounds and gain a bit of energy along the way and, if you decide it's not for you, your beloved granola will still be waiting for you when you return. :)

DO I HAVE TO FOLLOW A PERFECT PALEO REGIMEN?

No! I have yet to meet a person that follows a perfect paleo diet. And I've been to all the conferences and eaten alongside several of the paleo celebs. Trust me: ain't nobody got time for perfect! If you want to really put paleo to the test though, I suggest that you try to follow it as closely as possible for those first 30 days just so you can accurately gauge how well it works for you.

Most of us in the paleo world abide by an 80/20 approach: 80% of the foods we eat are paleo and 20% of the time we allow ourselves treats that are not perfectly paleo. As long as you don't have any major intolerances, that approach seems to be the easiest to sustain long term. For me that means that when I go out with friends, I have white rice with my sushi or I'll have some organic corn chips to dip into guacamole, and perhaps a gluten-free slice of cake here and there. I'm very careful to remain gluten free 100% of the time since I react pretty violently to gluten as does one of my kids.

A note on autoimmunity: Sometimes straight out-of-the-box-paleo alone is not enough. If you've had an autoimmune disease for some time and your healing stalls or does not improve on a simple paleo diet, then you may want to look into an autoimmune paleo diet which further restricts nightshades, eggs, nuts and seeds, NSAIDs (like Ibuprofen) etc. Don't worry! The autoimmune protocol is usually a temporary elimination diet until you can figure out which of those foods you react to and which you're ok with.

CHAPTER 2

PALEO GROCERY SHOPPING

On the paleo diet, it isn't enough to just change which foods you eat.
You've also got to think about the source of the food.

When we first started out with paleo, we were shopping in our regular grocery stores and farmer's markets. We soon realized the importance of buying pastured meat directly from the farmer so as to make it more affordable and also support our farmers! After many months, we decided to purchase a small freezer so we could buy meat in bulk.

Recently we upgraded to an even bigger commercial freezer and now purchase whole animals from the farmers (who, by then, were also our friends). Not only is this more affordable, but it is also more environmentally friendly and supports the local economy. You can usually find freezers on Craigslist for $150–$200 and they'll save you much more than that in the long run.

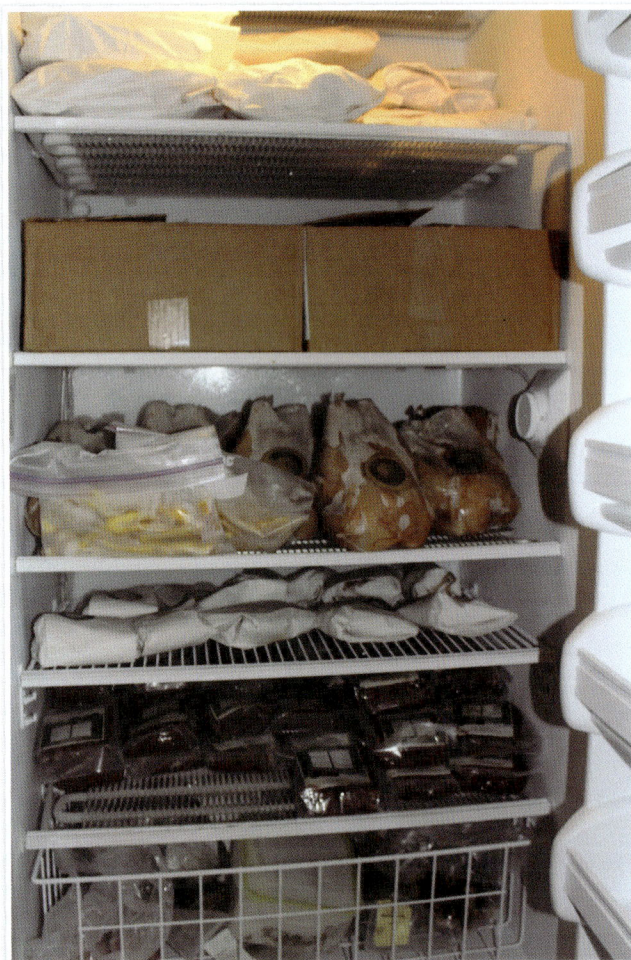

As you've probably guessed, meat is the biggest part of our food budget by far. Pastured meat usually costs about 50% more than conventional grain fed meat, although this varies quite a bit by location.

If you're just starting out, try to eat pastured and local foods as much as possible. But don't sweat it too much. You may need to make some compromises for budget or availability reasons and that's ok.

I've heard a few people say that they've thrown in the towel altogether because they're not able to find and/or afford perfectly pastured meat. As I mentioned in the previous section, *none of us eat a 100% perfect paleo diet*. Just take it one day at a time and do the best you can at each stage. You can upgrade as you are able.

PASTURED MEATS

You know the phrase, "you are what you eat"? Well, it doesn't just apply to humans! The quality of the meats we eat will vary depending on *what they ate*. Animals like cows, pigs, and chickens are NOT meant to be cooped up while eating grains fed to them by farmers. When out at pasture and eating the diet they were meant to eat, the animals become much healthier, and thus healthier to eat. Compared to "conventional" meats, pastured meats have much higher levels of healthy fats, B vitamins, vitamin A, vitamin E, and micronutrients like iron, zinc, and potassium[1]. To give you an idea just how much healthier pastured meats are, consider the fact that grass-fed meat contains about 4x more Omega 3 than grain-fed meat. The Omega 3 to Omega 6 ratio is also a lot better: 1:3 in grass-fed beef compared to 1:20 in grain-fed beef![2] And you know all those arguments against eating red meat? Well, they don't apply to grass-fed red meat because of how nutritious they are and loaded with healthy fats.

You can usually find pastured meat at Whole Foods or other specialty grocery stores. They usually only have a few cuts and it is definitely pricier than its grain-fed counterparts. However, lately some big-box stores like Costco have started carrying things like grass-fed beef as well! Prices will vary based on location.

The ideal place to buy your meats from would be your local farmers. Keeping your purchases local not only ensures freshness of your meats but also helps keep costs down, builds relationships, supports your local economy, and requires fewer resources like fuel to get the meat to you.

You can also purchase pastured meats online. The number of local farms offering online order and delivery services is increasing every day. You can find a nice list of them at my resource page.

Keep in mind that ALL meats are considered paleo. If it is accessible and you have it in your budget, then you may want to start experimenting with meats like ostrich, quail, duck, venison, and so forth. Since not everyone has access to these meats, I am only going to go over the more conventional options for meat.

Beef

I currently buy a whole cow at a time. I love supporting my local farmer this way and also love respecting the animal by eating "nose to tail". This also is the most economical way to do it as it brings the per-pound cost of the beef down significantly. When buying grass-fed beef, look for fatty cuts because they are a great source of Omega 3 and other healthy fats. But, if you are buying grain-fed beef, then it is better to opt for lean cuts. This is because the toxins (like all those growth hormones they give grain-fed cows) are stored in the animal's fat and then get passed into your body[3].

Lamb

We didn't eat much lamb at first because it can be very pricy. Then we started buying whole lamb from our local farmer, which brought the cost down quite a bit.

If you are eating out and want to stick to pastured meats, then lamb is usually your best bet when eating out. American lamb is grass-fed for most of its life but often is "grain finished", meaning that it is fattened with grain right before slaughter. Still, a much better bet than grain fed beef, which is what you will likely be served at a restaurant. Interestingly, Australian and New Zealand lamb are almost always grass-fed and finished.

Pork

In the paleosphere, bacon is something we often joke about because it is a gateway to the paleo diet. This might have something to do with the fact that we've all been told for years to fear and avoid bacon because of its saturated fats. Of course, everything we've been told about fearing saturated fat is wrong.

Saturated fat is essential for biological functions ranging from cell metabolism to hormone production[4]. And what about the myth that saturated fat will cause heart disease? *Saturated fat is actually important for protecting heart health*[5,6]. It reduces levels of a substance in our bodies called lipoprotein which is linked to heart disease. Saturated fat also increases HDL cholesterol levels (aka, the good cholesterol).

Despite the fact that scientific studies find no correlation between saturated fat and heart disease[7], the myth still continues. It's probably because it is easier to blame saturated fat than own up to the fact that all those unnatural, chemically-laden processed foods are to blame.

It may be tough to find pastured pork at your regular grocery store. We currently buy it from our local farmer. Visit http://www.eatwild.com/ to find a farmer near you.

Poultry and Eggs

Chicken is probably the meat we eat least often mostly because it is less nutrient dense and more expensive (if you're buying pastured) than the large ruminants I previously mentioned—and I'm more of a bang-for-my-buck kind of girl. We do like to have chicken about once a week. It is super easy to toss a chicken, veggies, and some herbs into a crock pot before leaving for work. It's easy and I come home to a ready-to-go bird. (see recipe on page 44)

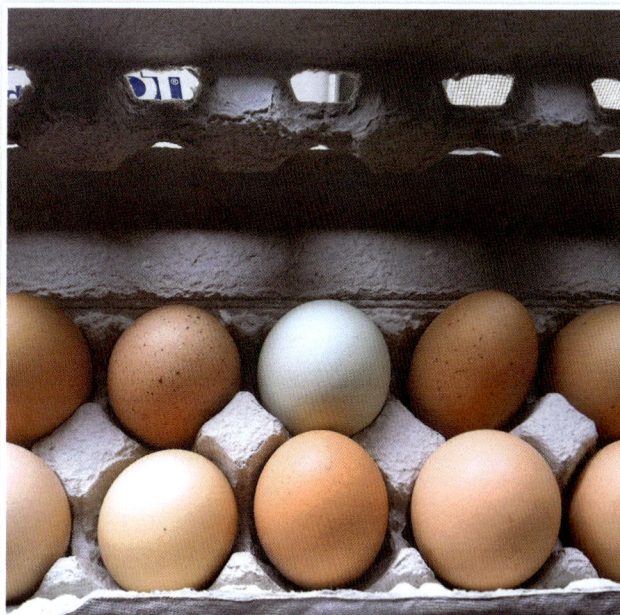

We buy whole chickens from our local farmer and free range eggs are delivered weekly from our CSA. You can buy chicken at Trader Joe's and Whole Foods, but it is very likely grain or soy fed (even if it says free-range and organic). BTW, chickens are NOT meant to be vegetarian. Along with seeds, they eat bugs and worms on pasture, and have even been known to eat bigger animals like lizards and mice. Of course, farmers do supplement their feed with grains and food scraps. This is perfectly fine. Pastured chickens will eat pretty much any plant when they can't find enough bugs, but ideally you want to make sure they are supplementing them with soy-free, GMO-free feed.

Fish

Wild caught fresh fish is ideal but we often have canned wild caught tuna, salmon and sardines. You can find wild caught fish seasonally at your local farmer's market. I like to stock up in my freezer when it's available and also love to have canned wild caught fish on hand for when we need a quick meal.

FRUIT AND VEGETABLES

It doesn't get more local than your backyard! If you're able to have even a small vegetable garden, that is ideal. You'll save some money, ensure your produce is organic, and get some vitamin D from the sun while you're out there!

We grow a few things in our garden but the bulk of our produce currently comes from our farm box deliveries twice a week. I highly recommend you sign up for a CSA (Community Supported Agriculture) in your area. Having produce show up at your door is one easy way to make sure you always have it on hand. To find a CSA in your area, you can visit Local Harvest, National Sustainable Agricultural Information Service, or AgMap.

If I need to buy vegetables at the grocery store where they've likely been shipped from afar, I often opt for frozen vegetables. The reason for this is that they are frozen at the peak of ripeness. By contrast, "fresh" produce is picked while it is still green and ripens on the truck on its way to the store. Since the produce isn't ripe, it doesn't have its full nutritional value or taste.

When you buy organic produce you are encouraging your farmers to grow organic. If you're not able to buy all organic produce I would prioritize by avoiding the "dirty" fruits and vegetables (the ones that are most heavily sprayed by pesticides) and instead opt for the "clean" fruits and vegetables (the ones which usually aren't heavily sprayed)[8].

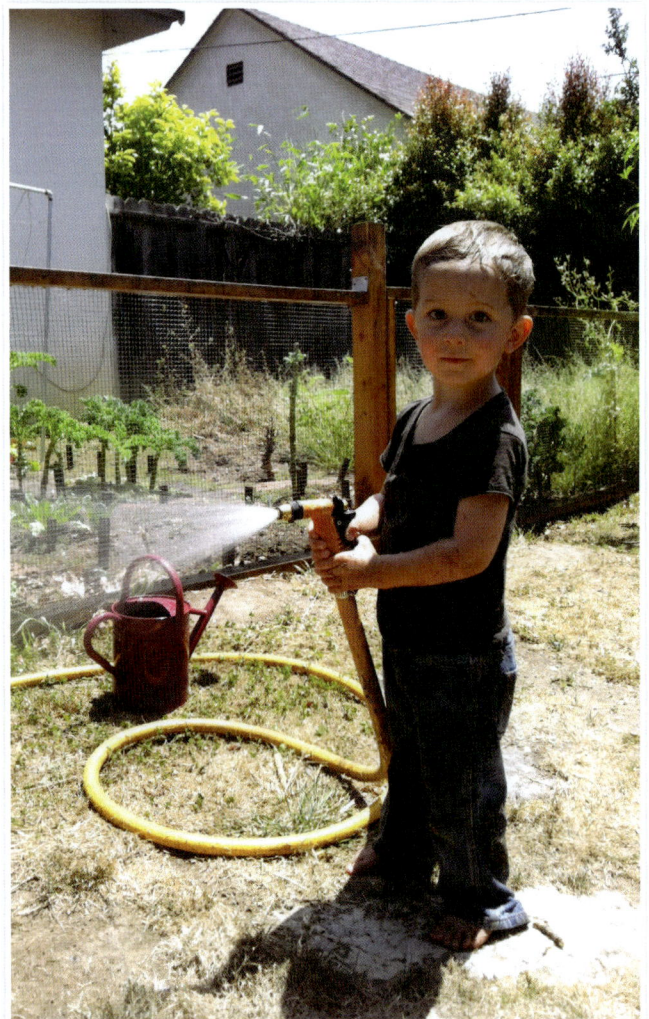

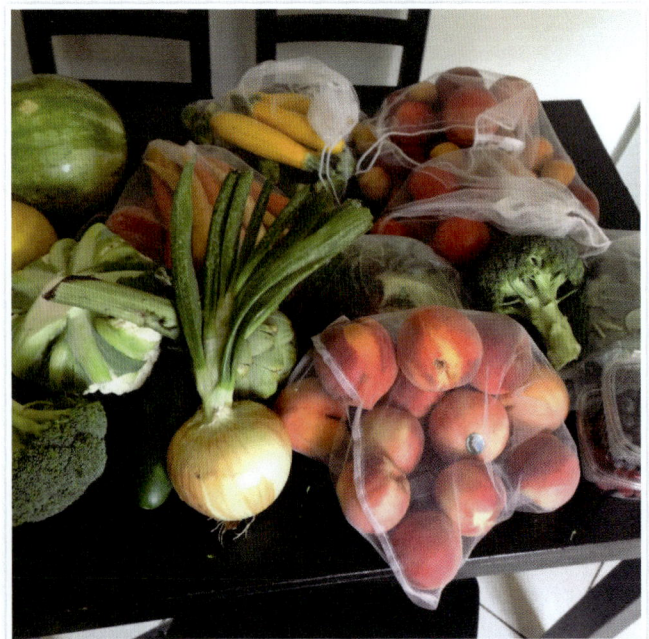

Paleo Made Easy: Getting your Family Started with the Optimal Healthy Lifestyle—with over 45 recipes!

Dirty Fruits and Vegetables	Clean Fruits and Vegetables
Apples	Asparagus
Celery	Avocados
Cherry Tomatoes	Cabbage
Cucumbers	Cantaloupe
Grapes	Eggplant
Hot Peppers	Grapefruit
Nectarines	Kiwi
Peaches	Mangoes
Potatoes	Mushrooms
Spinach	Onions
Strawberries	Papayas
Sweet Bell Peppers	Pineapples
Kale And Collard Greens	Sweet Peas
Summer Squash	Sweet Potatoes

FATS AND OILS

Paleo is most certainly NOT a low fat diet. Saturated fat is great for cooking as it is heat stable. Some of the delicious saturated fats you can use to cook with are:

- Coconut oil
- Ethically sourced palm oil
- Grass fed butter, if you tolerate dairy well (if not, try ghee!)
- Grass fed ghee,
- Pastured beef, pork, lamb, duck, or poultry fat

Unsaturated fats are best used for cold uses, such as salad dressings or pouring over food that has already been cooked. Heating unsaturated fats oxidizes them which causes free radicals to form while also killing the antioxidant properties of the fat. As you know, free radicals are the bad guys which damage cells and create a pathway for cancer, disease, and symptoms of aging. Since heating the oils also kills their antioxidants, you get a double whammy! It is much better to cook with saturated fats because they are more stable, which means that they aren't going to break down in the pan or on the shelf as easily or quickly.

If you do decide to cook with unsaturated fats, then it is best to opt for one with a high smoke point (the temperature at which the fat starts to burn and oxidation and free-radical formation occurs).

Some great unsaturated fats you can consume:

- Extra virgin olive oil
- Avocado oil
- Walnut oil
- Macadamia nut oil

The fats you want to *avoid* are the highly processed and refined fats that are commonly used at restaurants and in processed packaged foods. They're cheap, so they're everywhere. The most common forms of refined fats are butter substitutes like margarine, canola, and other seed oils.

The best part of paleo is being able to eat the *real*, full-fat delicious foods like butter that nourish our bodies instead of torturing ourselves with bland chemically-made substitutes that our bodies do not know what to do with.

NUTS AND NUT FLOURS

Nuts and seeds are great for their portability. I love to have nuts on hand to make trail mix for travel purposes but they are easy to overindulge in. Nuts are high in omega 6s, so take it easy! If you're just starting out, I wouldn't worry excessively about your nut consumption but, if you're goal is to lose weight and/or heal your gut, I would keep them to a minimum. Soaking and dehydrating nuts makes them easier to digest and more nutritious because it gets rid of some of the phytes[9].

Almond flour and coconut flour are probably the most commonly used wheat flour substitutes in the paleo world. I don't like to use them daily because I find it is easy to overindulge, but we do use them in our occasional paleo treats and they can be a life saver during the transitional period.

SWEETENERS

Going paleo doesn't mean we never indulge in treats and sweets. Of course it's always best to eat whole foods as found in nature and keep treats to a minimum. But, unless you live in a cave (pun intended), you'll likely benefit from having a list of unrefined minimally processed sweeteners you can use in your coffee, tea or baking.

My favorite sweeteners are:

- Raw honey, preferably local

- Grade B Organic Maple Syrup

- Raw organic sugar

I like to buy the honey at the farmer's market when available and I stock up on it since it does not expire.

Sweeteners to avoid:

- Aspartame

- Saccharin

- Sucralose

- Stevia (unless it's green leaf stevia)

These sweeteners were created in a lab. I don't know about you, but that's enough for me to stay away from them. Make sure to read labels since most *sugar free* products contain these chemicals.

For our baking products like coconut oil and almond flour, we purchase pretty much everything online. You can find the products I recommend on our resource page.

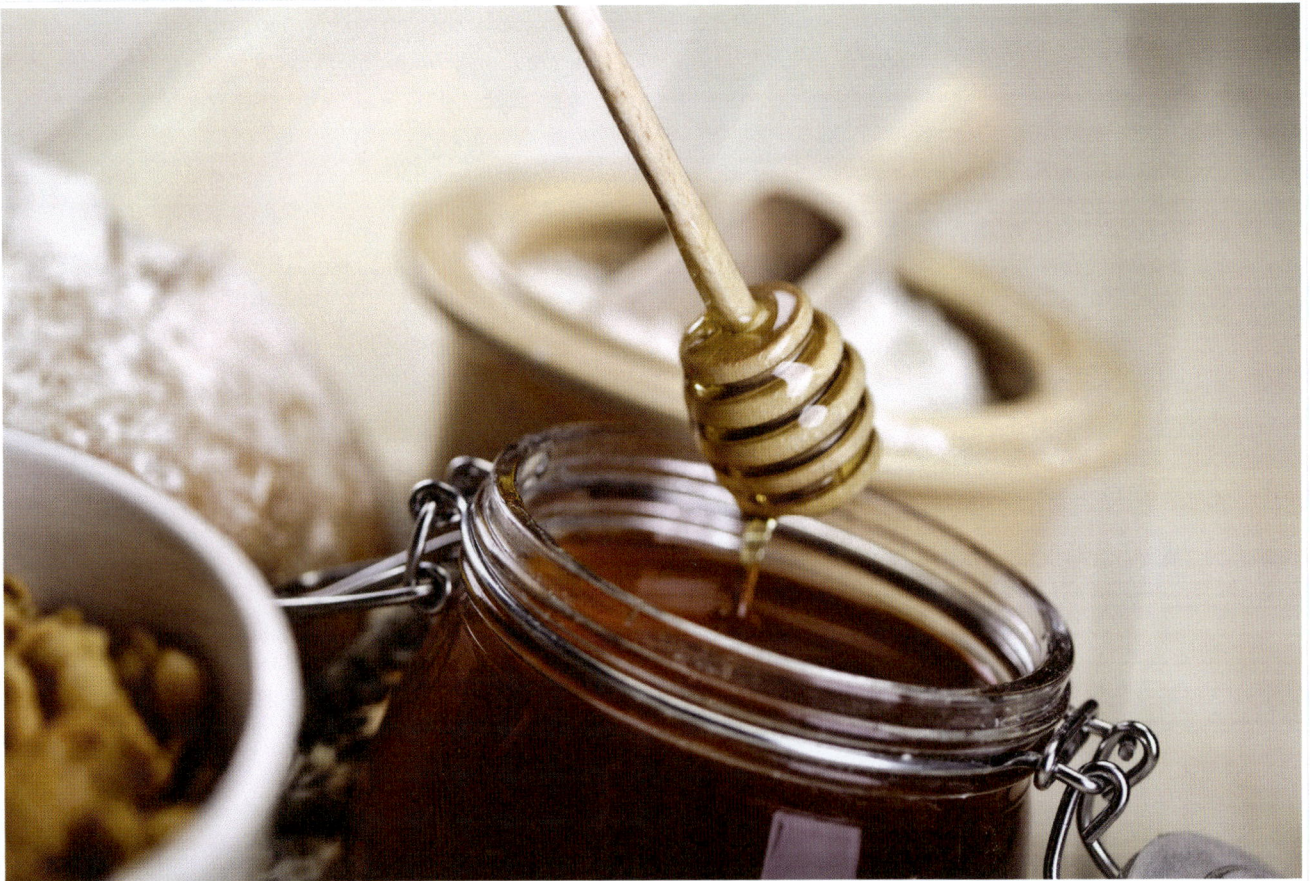

CHAPTER 3

PRIORITIZING PALEO

Making the room for paleo in your budget and schedule can take a bit of tweaking at first.

It is a commitment and it will likely mean making some sacrifices. I'm not gonna lie. For us the first 30 days were not easy. We were simply not used to spending so much time in the kitchen and spending so much money on food. Pasta was quick and cheap! Now we joke that we'd rather have a second freezer than a second car. Wait, actually that's not a joke at all...

DOES IT COST A FORTUNE?

It doesn't have to! When we first started transitioning to a paleo diet, we were eating pretty inexpensively. It wasn't easy to switch from buying beans and rice to buying grass-fed meat. So we had to make some compromises. For starters, we transitioned slowly. Then we also did some shifting in how we spend our time and money. It's all about priorities and sometimes sacrifices. If you can't afford pastured, organic, seasonal, etc. just do the best you can and upgrade when you are able.

I find that pretty accurate. "You get what you pay for" may be enough to explain this as well. If you can buy a lunch for $3 then, *yikes*, I don't want to know what's in that taco! Joel Salatin author of *Folks, This Ain't Normal,* summed it up very well when he said, "If you think Paleo is expensive you haven't priced out cancer lately". Can I get an amen?

Yes, You Can Afford Paleo!

When I started on the paleo road, it was clear to me that quality food costs more than we were used to spending. We decided quality was important and, since money doesn't grow on trees (darn!), we had to figure something out.

There are 5 of us. Only one of us earns a salary and let's just say it's not the salary of an investment banker. Did I mention we live in Los Angeles and spend almost half our income on rent?

But I still believe it is possible for everyone to afford paleo. Or, for that matter, to afford anything you want. It is all just about prioritizing.

I actually don't like to use the word "afford" since I truly feel that most of us can afford ANYTHING we want (within reason). We just can't afford EVERYTHING we want. In other words, some of us might say we can't afford an iPad whereas others might say they can't afford grass fed beef but pick up the latest iPad the day it comes out.

So here is how it whittles down:

1.   Make a budget and stick to it!

How many times have you heard that phrase? It's cliché, no doubt, but have you ever actually done it? And, if so, have you stuck to it? It doesn't really matter how much money we make if we are spending more than we're earning. It's what every corporation does and it's really as simple as adding and subtracting. Dave Ramsey explains it as putting "every dollar on paper on purpose" each month. I like Excel but really all you need is a piece of paper and a pen to record what comes in and what goes out. If you've never done this or it's been a while since you've done it, you might be shocked at how much money goes to each category.

2.   "If you fail to plan, you plan to fail" (Benjamin Franklin)

Menu planning is key for us. When we first started eating paleo we focused on meals which contain quality but less-expensive ingredients (like ground beef instead of filet mignon or kale instead of organic artichokes).

We did our planning by the week. We wrote out our 7 dinners and the ingredients we need for them (breakfasts and lunch are usually eggs, leftovers or salads), the couple treats we plan on baking, and any staples which are running low. Then we shop from that list. When we first transitioned to paleo there were no meal planning services. Now we save ourselves a lot of time by subscribing to Paleo Meal Plans.

3.   Buy in Bulk.

Everything is cheaper when you buy in bigger quantities whether you prefer to go to big box stores or order from online or local co-ops. The best part about buying in bulk is that you only have to do it once a month and then your weekly shopping trips can be quick and easy since the big stuff is taken care of. This not only works for non perishable items like toiletries, paper products, canned and packaged goods but can also work very well for buying meat in bulk as discussed

Paleo Made Easy: Getting your Family Started with the Optimal Healthy Lifestyle — with over 45 recipes!

in the previous chapter on page 14. You can also ask for discounts and you may be surprised to find out that you may even get a discount just for buying 4 or 5 lbs so a deep freezer is not necessarily a requirement.

4.   Spend Money on Whatever You Want!

No, that's not a typo. I guess I could say we've made sacrifices, but I'd rather see it as making choices on how we spend our hard-earned money. This will obviously be different in every household and we tweak things often as income fluctuates or as our needs and desires change along the way. For us food is our biggest expense after rent and we've made that expense a huge priority. We've decided that owning a home can wait; that we can make do with one car (that was bought used with over 100k miles, paid for in cash, and which we plan to run into the ground). When we first transitioned to paleo, we were grateful to have hand-me-downs and clothing swaps so that we could free up money to use on quality food. Even as our budget has increased over the years, we don't have cable or tablets and all our furniture except our mattresses and couch were bought on Craigslist. It is a numbers game at the end of the day and you have decide what categories are the most important for you to spend money on.

Finding the Time for Paleo

DO WE SPEND ALL DAY COOKING?

Sometimes! One day a week we try to do some batch cooking or food prep.

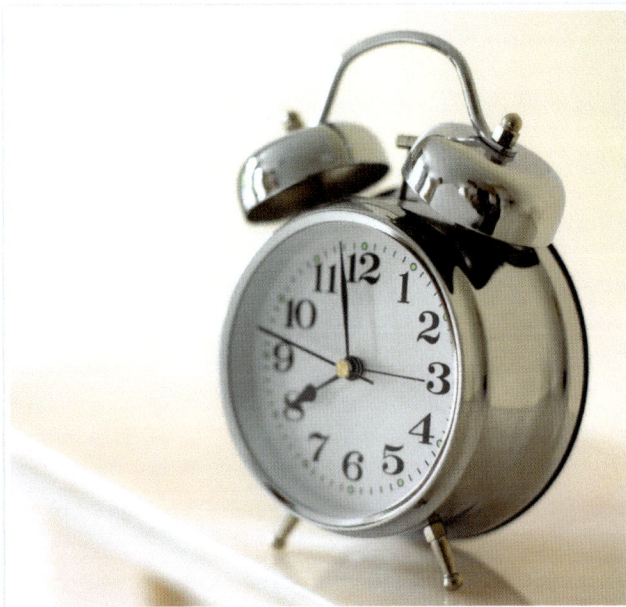

When we first made the switch to the paleo lifestyle one of the things we struggled adjusting to was how much more time it took each day to make real food versus boiling water for some pasta and opening a jar of pasta sauce. It felt like hours from prep to dishes. We soon learned that spending just a couple hours on a Saturday or Sunday would make the weekly meal prep a whole lot easier! It also saves dishes to be washed since I strategically use that food processor so it only needs to be washed out once or twice during the big cook fest. This is multi-tasking at its best!

Here's what I usually make during a day of mad kitchen prep on a weekend:

- 2 roasted chickens with vegetables
- braised kale (with bone broth) from our garden
- steamed broccoli
- ghee (from grass fed butter)
- grass fed beef burgers with hidden liver
- bacon (vanished same day, oh well)
- 2 gallons of kombucha (started for upcoming BBQ)
- chopped carrot sticks for snacks

I even taught an online cooking class on these prepping ahead techniques since I really believe it is one of the cornerstones of my success.

That sounds like a lot! But so many things can be done simultaneously that it really doesn't take more than a couple hours! Here is how it breaks down:

The night before
- Plan what you will be prepping if you haven't done so earlier in the week
- Set your frozen meats out to defrost

The cooking!
Start with the things that will take the longest to prep/cook.
I start by brewing tea for my kombucha. If you really want to batch it, brew several batches of it!
See page 59 for recipe and brewing instructions
While that is brewing and cooling, I get the chickens rinsed off and in the oven with potatoes or other vegetables. Use timers, they are your friends!
Then I place the butter in the pan to make the ghee and start the most hands-on task: the "Hidden Liver" burgers. Recipe on page 45.
While keeping an eye on the ghee and burgers, wash and cut up carrots for carrot stick snacks during the week!

Add one more pan with pastured bacon to cook up. Warning: if kids and canines are present, your chances of having leftovers are ZERO.

If you have another burner available, use it to steam some vegetables (I usually have all 4 burners going!)

Braise some kale or collard greens in bone broth. As the bone broth evaporates, the minerals are left behind. (Homemade Bone Broth recipe on page 65)

That's it! Several meals and snacks in just a couple of hours! Sip some kombucha while you're doing it and you've got yourself a little party!

Every few months it seems we evolve (pun intended) to fit our life as it changes. Sometimes that means having macadamia nuts and raisins in the diaper bag for a hectic afternoon; other times it means challenging ourselves to eat more organ meat or fermented foods each week to take our health up a notch. Most of the time, we just try to fit as much real food into our real world life as possible. And, every once in a while, we resort to ordering a gluten free pizza because life gets crazy sometimes. That's our 20%

Cavemen had nothing else to do than seek, prepare and consume food all day, every day between naps. That's obviously not the life we live. Most of us have jobs; kids have activities to be shuffled to, and somewhere in the midst of all that, we all have to eat.

It is possible to eat a paleo diet and have a busy life. At least 80% of the time. I promise.

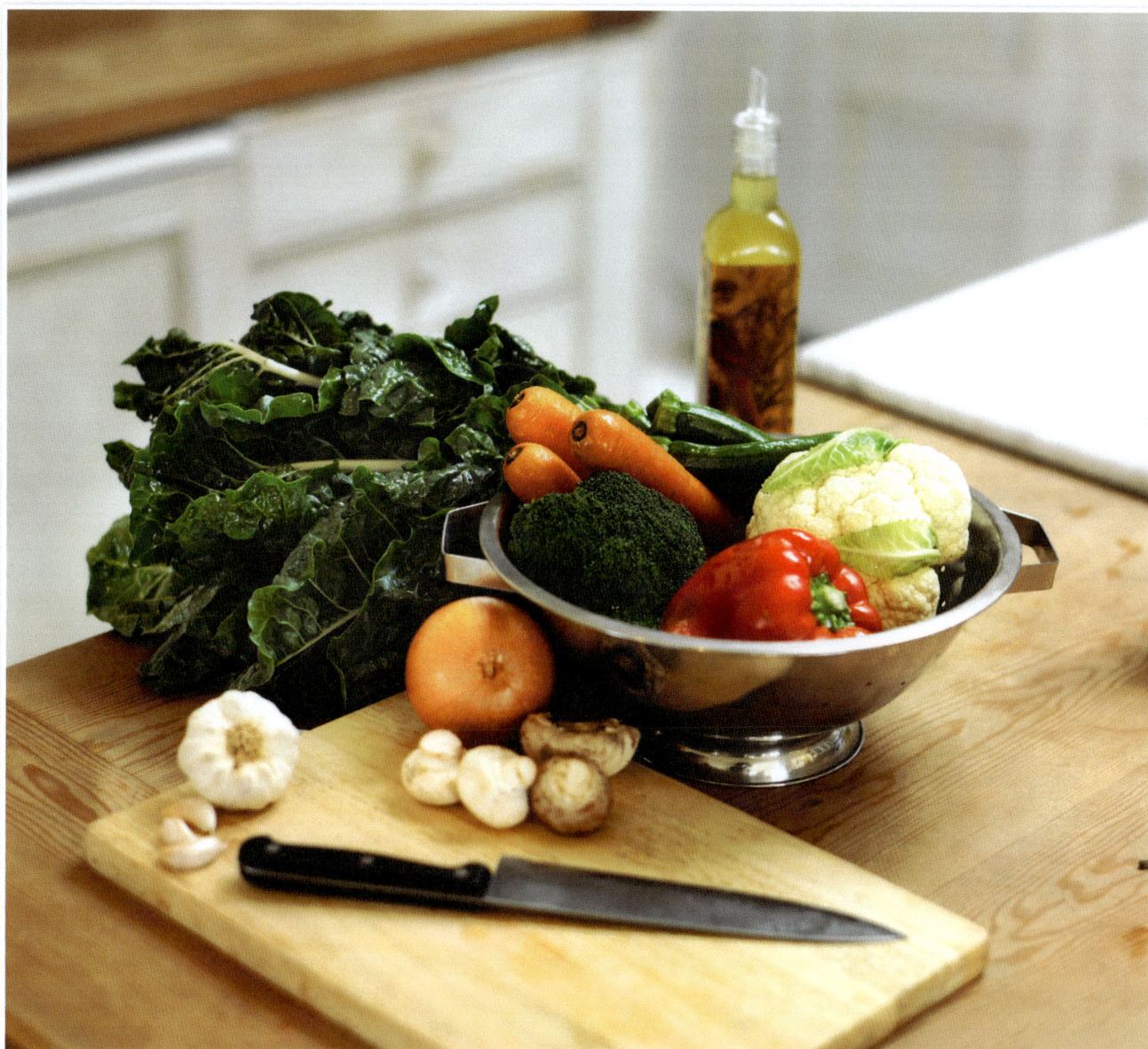

CHAPTER 4

TRANSITIONING YOUR PALEO FAMILY

Chances are, if you're anything like me, once you adopt a paleo lifestyle
and start experiencing life changing results there's not shutting you up.

You want your friend, your cousin, your co-workers and the stranger on the street to embrace paleo. You think it will solve global warming and bring world peace. So, it's only natural that you'll *at the very least* want those closest to you, in your own house, to follow this lifestyle as well. But how can you help them? Well, for starters if you want to help the stranger on the street I suggest you start a blog. Grabbing strangers by the shoulders and shaking them is apparently assault, or maybe it's battery. Either way, I don't recommend it. But let's talk about those closest to us...

RELUCTANT SPOUSES

I get this question a lot: *"How can I get my spouse to eat paleo? He/she keeps bringing cookies into the house and it's driving me crazy!"*

The short answer is... you can't.

For the sake of simplicity, I will use "he" and "him" in this section, although this could just as easily apply to a wife or girlfriend.

If your husband thinks you've fallen off the deep end with this paleo thing as my husband did when I first started, just know you're not alone. You've got to admit, wouldn't this have sounded insane to you a few years ago too? Sure, it worked for your friend so-and-so but do we all have to give up our cereal in the morning?

Living with someone who now eats very differently to you is not easy. Food is a big part of daily life! We eat three times a day and attend social events that are heavily focused on food. But, you obviously can't force anyone to eat the way you do if they don't want to. So, what can you do to help get your spouse on board?

How to Help Your Spouse Embrace Paleo

1. Lead by Example

If acquaintances are coming up to you telling you how great you look, or how happy you look, or how much better you or your kids are performing, you'd better believe he's noticing as well. Give it a few weeks of simply letting him see how this lifestyle is changing your body, mood, and life. His interest will pique.

2. Do the Shopping and Cooking

If you've always done the shopping and cooking, great! Just keep at it, but with paleo ingredients. If he's the one who has always done it or you've shared the task, offer to take over! Yes, it will be more work if you have a reluctant spouse, but it's just a few weeks during the transition that making it easier for him is really important. A few shifts will be easy and either go unnoticed or, at the very least, will likely not result in any resistance. For example, swapping out the margarine for delicious grass-fed butter or ghee or switching from grain-fed to grass-fed beef. If ditching all bread and pasta will cause a ruckus, perhaps switching to gluten-free alternatives will be a good bridge towards paleo for him. No, they don't taste the same, but it is something you can experiment with and see if it is helpful for him to occasionally still have these favorites. Ask him what he'd like to eat and paleoify his favorite foods. Pack his lunches! Also, if there's ever a time for paleo treats, it's during the transition. I remember relying on treats more than I do now because sometimes you just need a paleo muffin or brownie to keep yourself from losing your mind.

3. Pick Your Battles

Does he absolutely live for corn chips and salsa on Friday nights? Let him have them! It's not about being perfect. You can still experience many benefits of paleo without following it like a religion. Most people are paleo 80% of the time and, as an adult, he'll ultimately have to decide what his 20% is if he even wants to do this.

*Paleo Made Easy: Getting your Family Started
with the Optimal Healthy Lifestyle—with over 45 recipes!*

4. Offer New Things One at a Time

Sometimes *you* think he'll never give up this or that, but it's just because he doesn't know there's an alternative that is healthier and also delicious. I'm not saying to swap his potato chips for a carrot stick, but perhaps you can upgrade his potato chips to some which use avocado oil instead of rancid canola oil. You can also introduce new things simply by having them around. Sometimes it ends up being an interesting experience. I found this out at work. I happened to have kale chips and, to be polite, offered them to a colleague who I would have bet money would say no and/or hate them. Turns out he's now a kale chip addict. Who knew?

5. Be Patient.

You likely didn't hear about paleo one day and jump in with both feet the next. Why would he? For some people, cold turkey is just not the best approach. Changing one thing at a time is easier for some people. Just keep doing your thing. For my husband, I think one of the things that helped was hearing it from a guy. I'd show him the success stories from guys on Robb Wolf and Mark Sisson's websites, and those were much more relevant to him than female success stories. Ask him if he'll go to a local paleo meetup so he can hear the success stories first hand. It's interesting to see how the once-resistant spouse goes on to chat with all the other paleo dudes about how great they all feel. Mission accomplished ;)

KIDS AND PALEO

Eric and I often get asked how we get our kids to eat paleo, or get comments on how lucky we are that our kids will eat "this stuff". I assure you, it's not luck.

Let's rewind for a minute...

When I first started paleo, I did it solo. I did it because I thought I was the only "broken" one in my house, with health issues that required this extreme elimination diet. Some days, that meant we were all eating beautifully (paleo-ish); other days it meant I was scavenging in the kitchen for something I could eat while Eric and kids had pizza delivered (Folks, don't try this at home while you're transitioning...it was torture).

A month into it, with more health improvements than I could count and a lot of reading under my belt, it was very clear to me that Sofia, who was then 3 years old, would very likely benefit from removing gluten and possibly dairy from her diet. Eric humored me and we removed gluten from the house, making the commitment to do it for 30 days. By week two, the behavioral and health improvements in the kids were undeniable and, by accident, Eric was feeling great as well. **We were sold.**

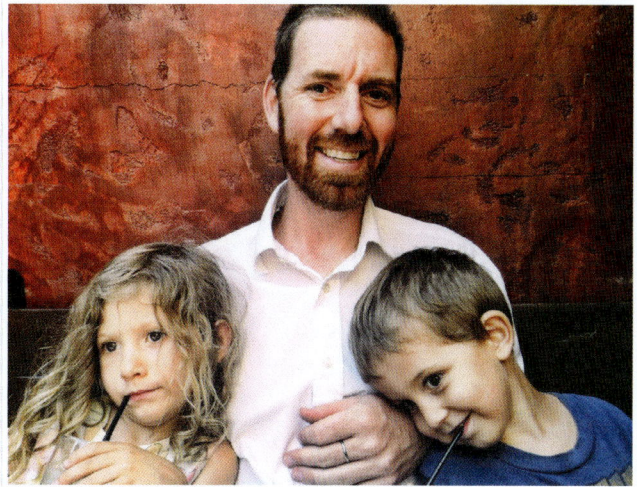

Before we started this journey my kids diet consisted most days of the following so-called "healthy" foods: Oatmeal for breakfast with raisins and slivered almonds, quesadillas for lunch with whole wheat tortillas and organic cheese, and maybe some grilled chicken breast, pasta with Bolognese, or beans and rice for dinner. Sprinkle in fruits and a few vegetables throughout the day, and that was our diet. We ordered pizza and/or ate out about once a month, mostly for budget reasons and also for "health".

We thought we were doing everything right, but were still overweight, tired, and got sick often. The kids were tired and cranky too and they got sick several times a year.

I knew the transition might not be easy, but it was a challenge I was willing to take on.

Three important things we learned during these first few weeks:

- Kids will not starve to death if you don't have the junk they want

- Kids will eat whatever you put in front of them if you hold your ground long enough and firmly enough

- Kids are unbiased when it comes to foods that we adults, with our biased preconceived notions, think are "weird" (ie: organ meat, fermented food etc)

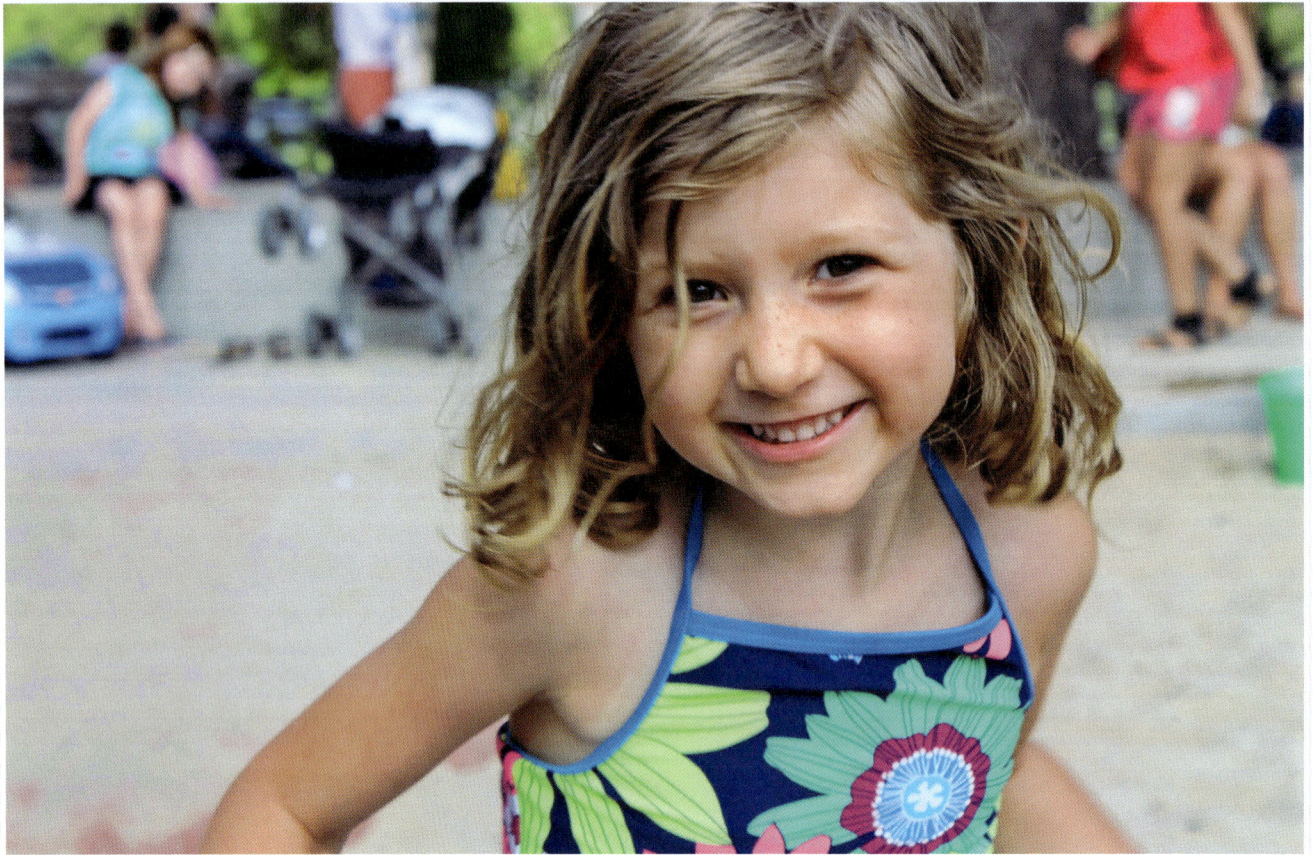

How to Transition Your Kids to a Paleo Diet

1. Start Slowly:

Swap out one food or meal at a time and let them adjust. When we first transitioned the quesadilla junkies, I just swapped out the tortillas for their gluten free counterparts (brown rice tortillas from Trader Joe's) and also reduced the frequency of their rotation in the menu (twice a week instead of 4–5 times per week). I focused on remaining gluten free 100% of the time and swapping out one non-optimal food at a time as we ran out of it.

2. Run Out:

Just run out of stuff and just don't buy it again. Don't take them to the store if that's a problematic trip during that transition period. At first, our kids asked for oatmeal every morning. Some days we just told them we ran out and told them all we had was eggs. We lied.

3. Pick Your Battles:

For me the most important thing is that the kids remain gluten free. If we're out to eat or at a friend's house, I let the kids eat treats so long as they are gluten free. When my mom or mother-in-law watch the kids, the only thing we request is that they remain gluten free and, of course, we also leave the fridge stocked with plenty of paleo foods that will be easy for them to reheat and serve. Is a gluten free cookie still just a cookie? Yes it is and many of the ones you will find at the store are loaded with even more junk than their regular counterpart, but we don't have to be perfect to experience the health benefits of paleo and so far the only thing that my kids can't tolerate even a bite of is gluten.

4. Hold Your Ground:

I hear from a lot of parents that "little Johnny just won't eat anything but (insert junk of choice here)". Actually, he will.

If you're ready to make changes and you believe the food your kids eat is not what is best for them, then just say NO. Then stick to it just like you do in other parenting scenarios that are not negotiable (running into the street, seatbelts on in the car, you get the gist).

Our kids definitely noticed each change we made. Some days we got a mini hissy fit. Other days we were boycotted. Other days we got a full on kicking-on-the-floor fit (which, of course, we filmed for blackmailing later in life).

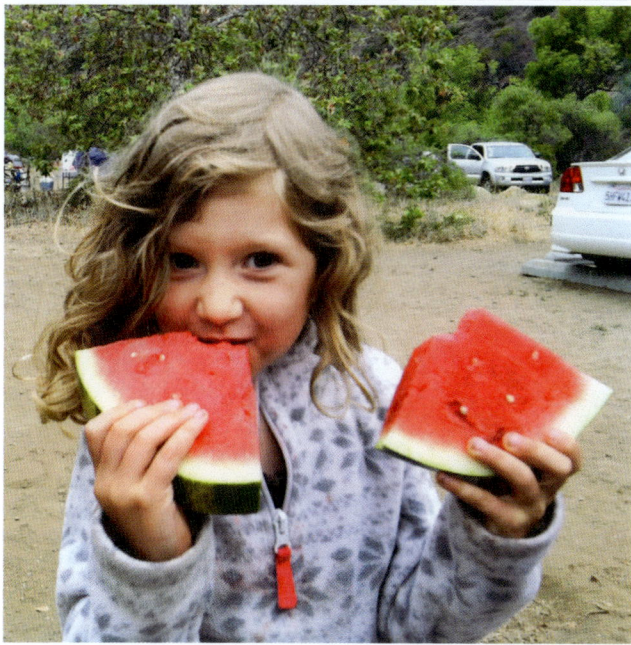

I'm not saying this is going to be easy but my guess is that if you're reading this chapter it will be worth the trouble.

5. Experiment with Traditional Superfoods:

The coolest thing about grabbing them while they're young (ha! that sounds like we're pushing drugs or something) is that they don't have peer pressure or preconceived notions working against them. Our palates are pretty messed up after many decades of hyper-palatable foods but theirs are a lot more malleable. They don't mind liver, fermented cod liver oil, and other "crazy" things. Before I could stop her, Sofia was gnawing on chicken feet like it was the best thing ever. And I was loving it because I knew that those chicken feet from our pastured, local chicken farm were full of bone building gelatin, vitamins, and minerals to feed her growing little body.

So, it's not luck. It's persistence. And laziness.

I often, somewhat jokingly, describe my parenting style as lazy. Sometimes that happens to coincide with some attachment parenting type stuff: breastfeeding, baby led weaning, baby wearing... But really, it is mostly an outcome of laziness. I have 3 kids and I'm 14 years into this parenting gig. That's a lot of sleep deficiency and parenting books read. For my first, I may have played "short order cook" for a stint. By my third, that just wasn't going to happen. Mama's tired!

The transition won't happen overnight but it will go a lot faster than you think. It also doesn't have to be perfect. We are far from it and honestly have no interest in being paleo perfect. As they feel better, it will get easier, and there will also be more motivation to stick with it.

Do my kids still whine and beg for food, especially treats? Yes, they do (relentless little people). But now those "treats" they ask for are usually kombucha, fruit, bacon, and definitely any baked paleo treats if they're around. We joke that we have to hide fruit and nut bars like they're contraband around here.

PALEO FROM A TEENAGER'S PERSPECTIVE

Now, teenagers are a whole other ball of wax. On the one hand, you can reason with them (ok, not always, but more than you can with a 2 year old). On the other hand, you're a little less in control of the food they eat, especially if they're at school, out at the mall, or at friends' houses. Like with any area of parenting a teen, you'll have figure out what works for your family. We found value in giving her the time and space to figure out a few things for herself. We only requested that she not eat things we were trying to keep the little ones away from in front of them so as not to have that battle to deal with. The rest of the time, we tried to remain as non judgmental as possible, even as she would race straight to the bathroom when she would come home from hanging out at the food court with her friends.

I interviewed my oldest daughter who is 14 and this is what she had to say about her experience with Paleo so far:

How long have you been eating paleo?
Probably about 9 months—a year.

What did you eat prior to your family finding this lifestyle?
Well, even before we went paleo, my family was always considered "healthier" than my other friends. Especially because one night I had so much spinach (not by choice) that my tongue turned green. It was hard to get my normal color back. I was eating a peanut butter and jelly sandwich every day for lunch at school but it was with whole wheat bread (which we found out isn't as healthy as we thought) and after school I had one sliced tomato with salt and oregano (I still do!), we had pasta sometimes and pizza (yum!). It's a little bit hard to remember what we ate. I mean, I focus so much on the things that are my favorite foods that it's hard to remember the stuff I don't like as much.

What is your favorite food?
During the transition, my favorite foods didn't change but now I just can't eat them very often. Like cheese pizza, French

Paleo Made Easy: Getting your Family Started with the Optimal Healthy Lifestyle—with over 45 recipes!

fries, my dad's homemade chocolate chip cookies, bread, Honey Nut Cheerios, corn empanadas, quesadillas and tortellini.

What do you do when you go out with your friends to the food court at the mall?

Most of the time I just get whatever I want. But the times when I was being more strict with myself I got frozen lemonade and French fries.

Do you notice a difference when you eat SAD (Standard American Diet) food?

Well, I get more cranky and my acne gets A LOT worse!

What would you say is the hardest thing about eating real food?

Probably the amount of organ meat. I like meat but I'm pretty picky about it. Also, when I go to my friend's house for a sleepover, the food that used to fill me up until the next meal time barely holds me for an hour. It turns me into an eating machine. In the end I feel full, but empty. Like full of food, but empty of nutrients that make me feel...relaxed. You'll understand if you experience it.

Would you say you're an 80/20 (80% paleo/20% non paleo), more or less?

Yes. I eat paleo at home but on the weekends when I go out I choose what I want. Recently I've been 100% paleo to prepare and recover from my surgery but after 5 more months I'm going back to my old ways.

What changes have you noticed since adopting this lifestyle?

I noticed that when I eat clean my acne goes away. Just vanishes. It's pretty amazing actually. And sometimes I put coconut oil on my face, which also helps. With that combo, my face is softer than all my friends who have their fancy moisturizers.

Do you think you'll continue eating this way when you're an adult? Why or why not?

I don't think I can decide right now. I can barely decide what I want to wear to the mall. I think I'll probably be 80/20 because I know the dangers how gluten and dairy affect me but on the other hand, it's so hard to resist.

What would you say to another teenager who is thinking about going paleo, whether for weight, health or clearer skin? Is it worth it or should they run the other way?

I think it's worth it but I know it's really hard so I would say try your best and see the results YOU get. Everybody's different. Besides, you don't have anything to lose, and you can always let yourself have a treat!

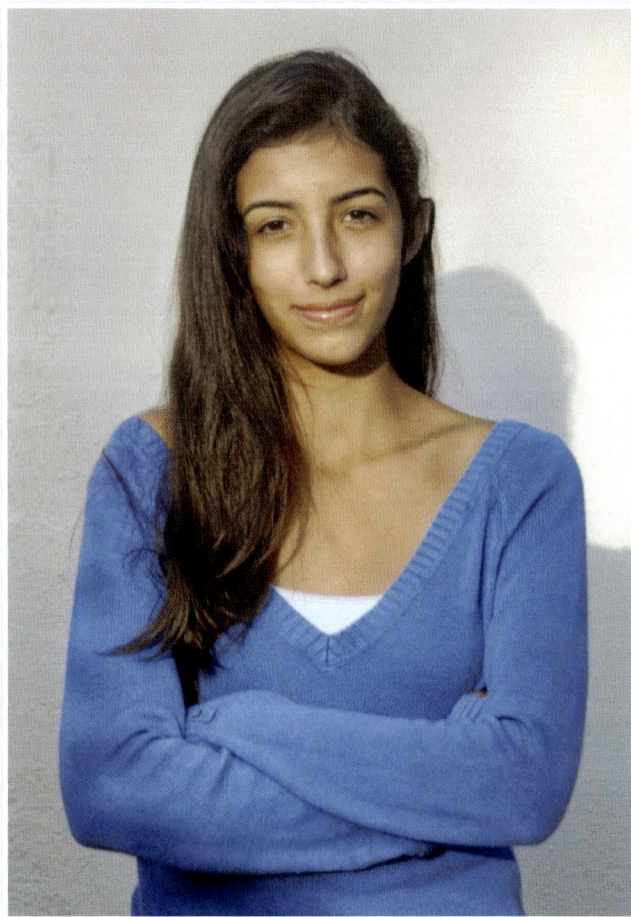

CHAPTER 5

PALEO IN TIMES OF ILLNESS

So what happens when you get sick?
Can you still eat Paleo when you're under the weather, in the hospital or recovering from major surgery?

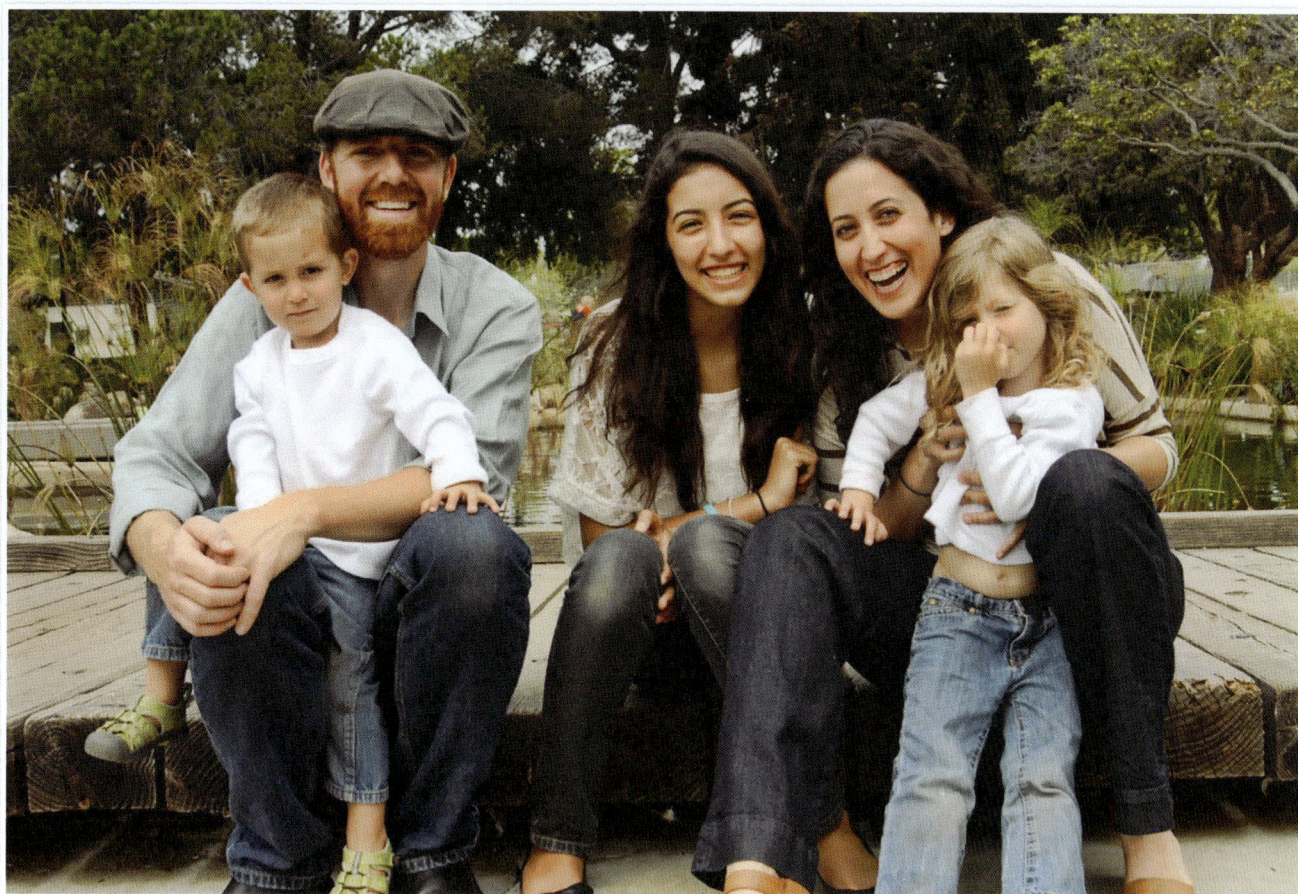

During times of illness, it is even *more* crucial to feed your body the nutrients it needs and craves so that it can to repair itself and thrive.

But, the truth is that when you adopt a Paleo diet you'll notice you very rarely get sick! During the first few months of transitioning the kids, I remember noticing how many of the preschool-wide bugs seemed to skip right over them! Now, the kids don't get a cold or flu (or worse) every other month as is common with preschoolers. They catch a cold about once a year and it lasts about 4 days instead of 10. If they get a fever, it lasts one day instead of 3. This is because their immune systems are strong and their little bodies have all the nutrients they need to fight back and keep things at bay.

Of course, this has to do with more than just food. Proper sleeping schedules, routines, and environment are all crucial for immune function. I also keep harsh antibacterial cleaners out of our home since living in a less-than-sterile environment helps build up the immune system so that it can protect the body as needed.

I used to catch every bug that came within a mile of me and was sick multiple times a year. I even had Epstein-Barr virus several times because my immune system was so run down. Stress management and nutrient dense food is an amazing combo.

*Paleo Made Easy: Getting your Family Started
with the Optimal Healthy Lifestyle—with over 45 recipes!*

WHAT TO DO IF YOUR KIDS ARE FEELING SICK

This is the time to take the nutrient density up a notch! This is the best time to prepare organ meat, gelatin, and broths.

Organ Meat

Hey, I'm a former vegetarian so I know exactly the face you're making as you read this right now. The thought of organ meat used to gross me out as well! But this is a cultural taboo that you should get over for the sake of your health. Organ meat is one of the most nutrient-dense foods you can eat. Compared to the muscle meats which we normally would eat, organ meat has 10 to 100 times more nutrients. They contain mega amounts of B vitamins (which are really important for your mental health and energy levels), iron, magnesium, copper, zinc, vitamin D (which is really important in winter), healthy fats, and more[10,11].

Of all organ meats, liver takes the prize. Not only is it one of the most nutritious of the nutritious organs, but it is generally pretty easy to find and cheap to buy. To give you an idea of how healthy liver is, check out this nutrient comparison[12]:

	GROUND BEEF (100 GRAMS)	BEEF LIVER (100 GRAMS)
Protein	23 grams	29 grams
Fat	16 grams	5 grams
Iron	2.4mg	6.5mg
Calcium	37mg	6.0mg
Magnesium	20mg	21mg
Zinc	5.8mg	5.3mg
Copper	0.1mg	14.3mg
Selenium	19.2mcg	10.1mcg
Vitamin A	0 IU	31718 IU
Vitamin B12	2.4mcg	70.6mcg
Folic Acid	10mcg	253mcg
Niacin	5.0mg	17.5mg
Vitamin B6	0.3mg	1.0mg

Keep in mind that these nutritional facts can vary depending on whether the animal was pastured (much healthier!), the age of the animal, and where it was raised. But, as you can see, organ meat is much richer in many hard-to-get nutrients.

If you think your kids or spouse will freak out at the thought of eating organ meat, check out my recipe for Hidden Liver Burgers on page 45. They'll never know! ;)

If you just can't stomach the thought of eating organ, there are capsules you can buy that are made from desiccated liver. I keep those on hand at the office when it's been a few days since my last organ meat consumption, since life can get unexpectedly hectic or stressful.

If anyone is under the weather or has had less than ideal sleep for whatever reason, I also like to double the Fermented Cod Liver Oil dose that we all take daily for a few days to help the immune system do what it needs to do. You may also want to consider increasing your vitamin D dose during that time and even including something like colloidal silver in your repertoire. Please consult with your naturopath or pediatrician to help figure out what supplements and doses are right for you.

Grass Fed Gelatin

Now, we are NOT talking about the junk gelatin you often see at the store full of additives, chemicals, and made from god-knows-what. As with anything, read the ingredients and if you have to start researching them, chances are you shouldn't eat it. If you don't recognize the ingredients, your body won't either.

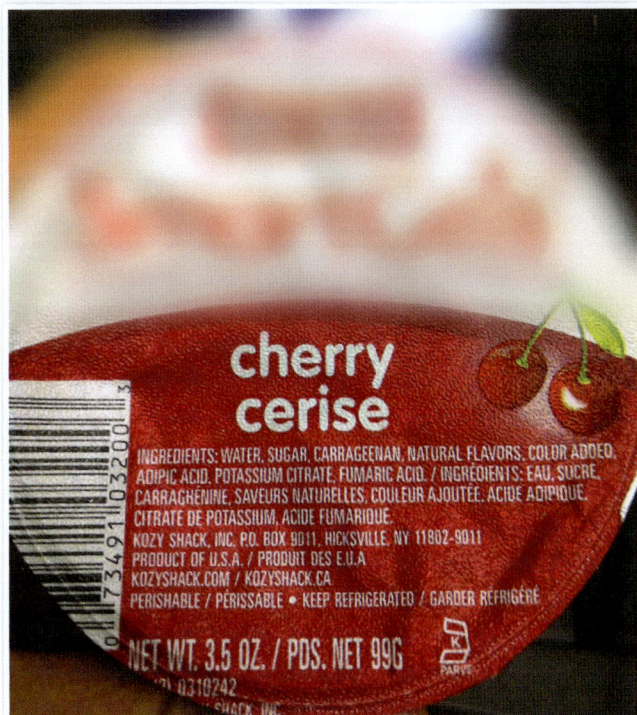

Real gelatin is made from the collagen found in bones and connective tissues of pastured animals. Gelatin is rich in the amino acids glycine and proline which are anti-inflammatory, hence why gelatin has been hailed as a natural remedy for arthritis.

Since gelatin is made from collagen, it is no surprise that it is great for your bones, joints, hair, skin, and nails. FYI, you can NOT absorb collagen through the skin, so all those collagen skin creams are useless. If you want toner skin, then the best way to get collagen is to take it from within. That's right, you'll have to eat your botox[13]. (wink)

The amino acids in real gelatin are also great for the liver and do wonders for detoxifying the body. It is also great at healing leaky gut[15].

This is an easy superfood to consume too! Kids and adults alike will love the gummies and jello recipes on page 83.

If you're in a hurry or have no energy, just dissolve a teaspoon or so of gelatin in your tea or soup and knock it back.

While my daughter was recovering in the hospital, I snuck in a bit of gelatin powder every chance I got. After all, gelatin is basically ground-up bone from pastured animals. Can you think of anything better to consume when you're actively trying to rebuild and repair bone?

BONE BROTH

Chicken soup has been the go-to remedy for illnesses for centuries. It earned its reputation for a reason! Now, we aren't talking about the junky stuff you can find in a can at the store. Real chicken soup is made the carcass of a whole chicken, which means it also contains gelatin. Making gelatin-rich bone broth is very easy: you basically just cook down the bones of pastured animals and voila! The resulting bone broth is rich in the minerals that your body needs to fight illness, and the nutrients are easy to absorb. It also supports red blood cell production[14]. Since gelatin helps detox the liver, it is also going to help you flush out your sickness quickly.

Bone broth shouldn't be reserved for times when you are sick. I try to drink a cup of bone broth 3–4 times a week since it is very beneficial for gut health and detox. I just put it in a coffee travel mug and sip it at work and at home.

I consider it my flu shot and botox in a cup. :)

SLEEP AND STRESS REDUCTION

Getting adequate sleep and keeping stress to a minimum is important to maintaining health but during times of illness and repair there is a definitely a good case for paying even more attention to these areas. Perhaps you can go to bed an hour earlier, postpone things that are not absolutely crucial this week, ask for help or take up meditation. For more on sleep and stress please see pages 35–37

AT THE HOSPITAL

When my daughter had major surgery on her spine and was going to be in the hospital for a week, I made sure to prepare an arsenal of healing foods. Many hospitals will include a mini fridge in the room. If yours doesn't than you can request one or see if they have one you can use in the parent's lounge or even nurses' lounge. Get creative! You can also buy a used fridge on Craigslist and resell it when you are done. Don't let something like fridge-accessibility get in the way of nourishing your loved ones when they need it most!

Paleo Made Easy: Getting your Family Started with the Optimal Healthy Lifestyle—with over 45 recipes!

When friends came to visit, I asked them to stop by my home where Eric was cooking up a storm and smuggle food to us at the hospital where all they seemed to have was low-fat processed foods.

It is sad really that you have to defend yourself in a place where you should be able to relax and know you are taken care of, but that's the reality.

Several times a day I offered her jello and soup made with gelatin-rich bone broth, avocado and fruit. I also made sure to have the nurses list on her chart that she's allergic to gluten and dairy. Allergies are taken quite seriously and luckily, by eliminating those two, most of the processed food goes out the window along with it.

Medications are beyond the scope of this book but I will also add that you may want to look into the different painkillers (acetaminophen, NSAIDs like ibuprofen, etc) and discuss with your doctors what is best for you in your particular case since they all have pros and cons.

The doctors and nurses were very impressed with how quickly and well Natalie was recovering and able to lift herself out of the hospital bed. Coincidence? I think not. The Crossfit she did leading up to surgery, her nutrient-dense diet, and carefully-selected supplement regimen set her up for success.

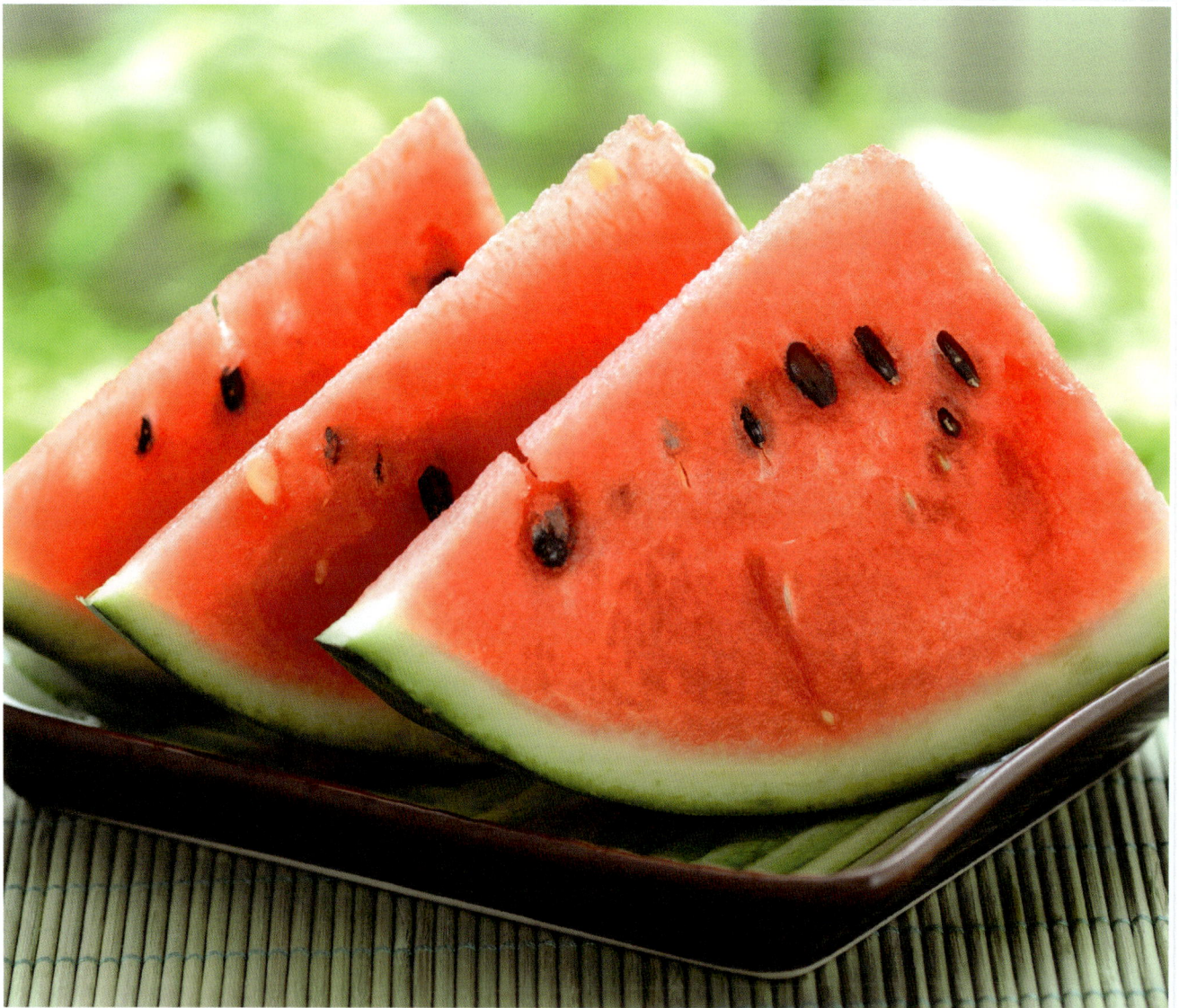

Paleo Made Easy: Getting your Family Started with the Optimal Healthy Lifestyle—with over 45 recipes!

CHAPTER 6

EATING PALEO ON THE GO

Is it possible to eat Paleo when you're a moving target? Business trips, vacation, and just plain life takes us out of our routine sometimes. If you think you have to toss the diet out the airplane window, think again!

The trick is to OVERplan and OVERprep.

As with any challenge, PLANNING is key. While there are always some curveballs that you can't plan for, there are many things you can count on and prepare for.

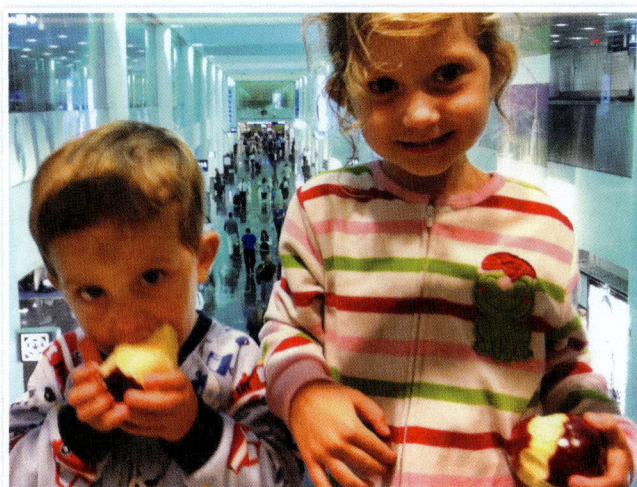

PALEO WHILE TRAVELING

In the last year alone, I've been on one international trip, 3 domestic plane trips, and several road trips. I managed to stick to my 80% paleo, 100% gluten-free lifestyle the entire time—and you can too! Although the food isn't always the same quality I have at home, I am able to get by just fine and haven't ever had to resort to a stale sandwich.

With my trips, I knew that:

- I would be on a plane twice each time
- plane delays are very likely if not expected
- plane food is not food at all
- I would be busy
- I would have no kitchen or cooking utensils
- if I didn't fuel my body well, I wouldn't be able to get the most out of the trip
- I turn into the wicked witch when starving

With this in mind, I made a list of all the foods that would keep well outside a fridge for several hours while traveling, making sure I had enough protein and fat since my body does not do well when those two macronutrients are lacking.

Examples of travel friendly food:

- hard boiled eggs
- carrot sticks (or other veg sticks)
- Larabars (or equivalent) containing fruit and nuts
- canned fish like tuna, salmon or sardines (buy packages or pop-tops, or pack a can opener)
- nuts (homemade trail mix with almonds and macadamia nuts)
- dried fruit
- coconut chips
- homemade jerky or store-bought if its gluten and soy free
- fruit like apples and bananas (if traveling internationally, make sure you consume them before going through customs to avoid a hell of a speech!)

Obviously, some of the above will need to be eaten or refrigerated sooner than others, so plan your eating accordingly.

And, yes, I get some looks at the airport when I bust open some fish—but I don't care! I try to eat it before boarding so the smell doesn't linger and I can dispose of it. People get on the plane with a bag of McDonald's food all the time and I find *that* obnoxious too.

Get Back on Track

As soon as you get home, get back to you usual routine and make sure to sneak in some extra nutrient-dense goodies like bone broth and fermented cod liver oil and some fermented foods like the recipes on page 58. You could also take probiotics for a few days to help your body get back on track.

PALEO WHEN EATING AT RESTAURANTS

Eating out when you have dietary restrictions is not always easy. Gluten seems to sneak into just about everything and most restaurants source their ingredients based on price, so the food quality can often be questionable. The more expensive the restaurant, the more accommodating and knowledgeable the staff will be and the better chances of the food quality being better. In any case, I'd rather eat out less often but go to a swanky place when I do. When I'm traveling, I'll often choose to stay somewhere with a kitchen and limit eating out to once a week. This makes it a heck of a lot easier to keep your diet under control, and also cuts back on restaurant expenses.

The best way to minimize a gluten exposure at a restaurant is to ask the waiters. Be incredibly specific with your questions, such as by asking, "is the fish dusted with flour?" or "does the sauce contain gluten?". Using phrases like "allergic to gluten" or even "celiac" will help them to understand the severity of your request. If your waiter doesn't seem confident ask him or her politely to double check with the chef. At first, you might feel like you are being a hassle or inconvenience, and it might be embarrassing to bring your own coconut aminos to the sushi place in order to avoid the wheat in the soy sauce but, for the sake of your health, it is most definitely worth the trouble and pretty soon it will be second nature.

Make Compromises

Unless you have to be on a super strict diet like the Autoimmune Protocol, you can probably handle relaxing your food standards just a tad so that you don't lose your mind while on the go. For instance, I usually don't eat fruit and nut bars or too many nuts. I did when I was first transitioning to paleo but nowadays I don't usually feel like I need a snack and I use fruit and nuts as treats. That said, I still bring several with me on my trips because I want an easy backup option in case I am hungry and having trouble finding something clean to eat. I usually only end up eating a couple of bars on my trips, but it is reassuring to know I have something to fall back on.

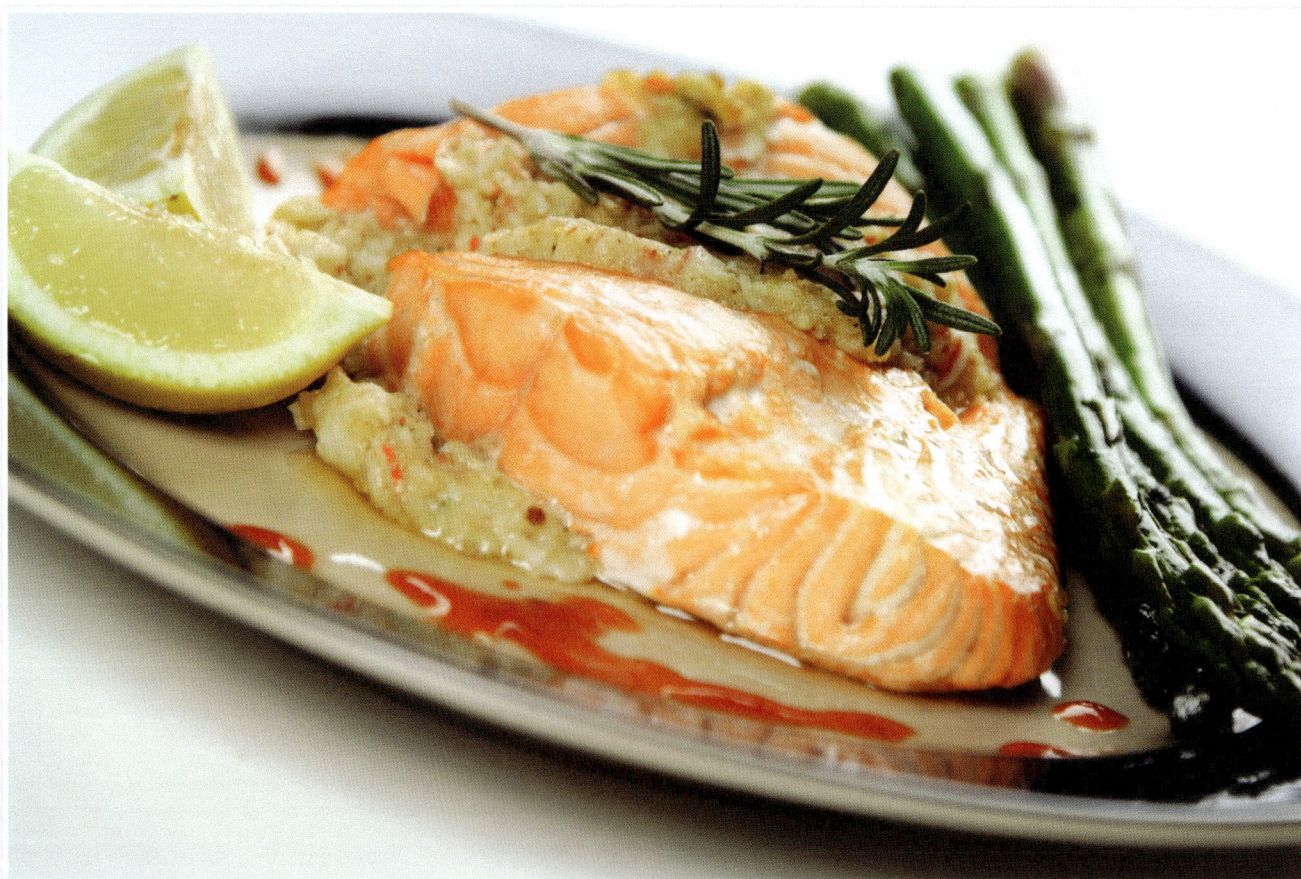

Paleo Made Easy: Getting your Family Started with the Optimal Healthy Lifestyle—with over 45 recipes!

CHAPTER 7

PALEO AT SOCIAL FUNCTIONS

One of the questions I often get asked is *what do you do when you attend social functions like a birthday party where the guests and hosts aren't paleo? How do you keep the kids away from the canola-oil-laden chips and gluten-filled cakes and snacks? How do you keep* **yourself** *from eating a bunch of junk?*

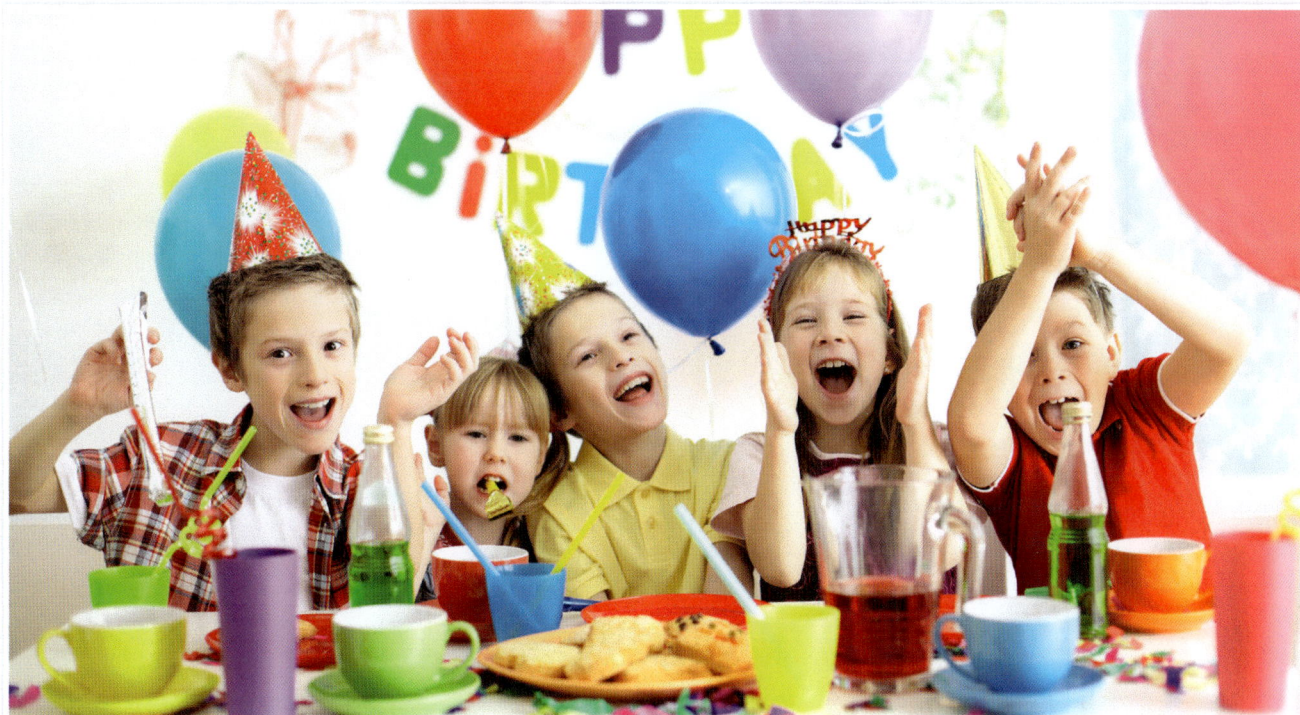

It depends!

When I first transitioned the kids to paleo, it was difficult. I was still trying to figure out what foods contained what ingredients, what they were sensitive to, what things were uber important, and which things I could let slide occasionally.

Over time, I learned that my 4 year old cannot tolerate gluten at all nor large amounts of dairy. My 14 year old is noticeably affected by gluten and dairy, but she is at an age where she is figuring that out for herself and I feel the need to step back and allow her to make her own food choices. In contrast, when my 3 year old manages to get his hand on some questionable foods before I can get to him, it doesn't seem to affect him too much.

As I've said before, we aren't paleo perfect. But that doesn't mean I let my 4 year old eat with abandon just because we are at a birthday party. That would absolutely wreck her. Instead, I make sure to plan ahead for the party and follow a few tricks.

PALEO TIPS AND TRICKS FOR ATTENDING A BIRTHDAY PARTY

1. Feed everybody before you leave the house!

I do this not only for parties, but also if I know I'll be out running errands for several hours. If everybody is well fed ahead of time, you'll simply eat less and/or make better judgments about food when it's placed in front of you. It's similar to the rule about not going grocery shopping when you're starving.

If our little adventure involves a long car ride, I even take something for us to eat on the way there, like beef jerky, homemade trail mix or a fruit and nut bar.

2. Take foods to share!

Talk to the host first and find out if you can bring some burgers or chicken to grill, a salad and a dessert to contribute!

Paleo Made Easy: Getting your Family Started with the Optimal Healthy Lifestyle—with over 45 recipes!

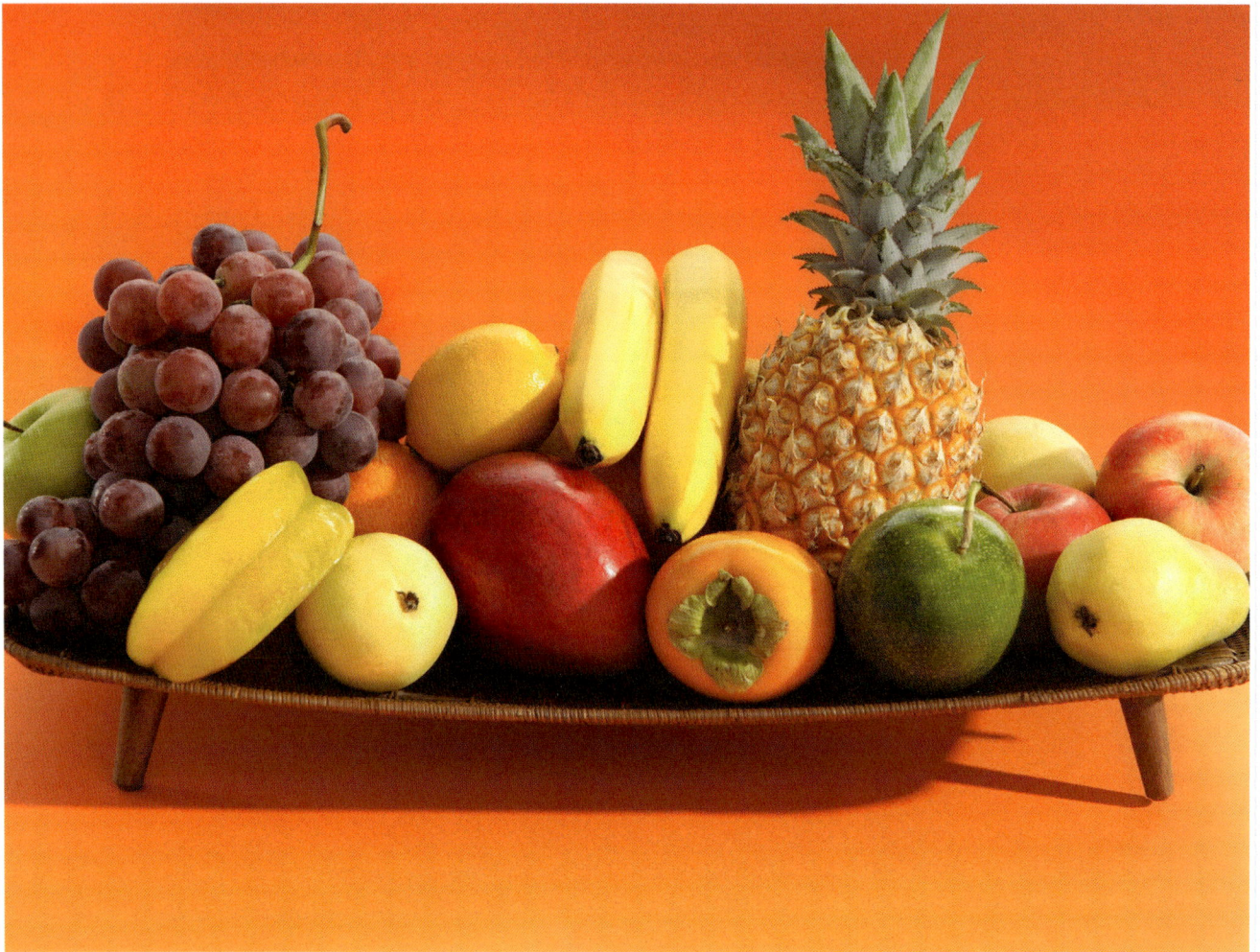

Chances are that food will be welcomed and that way you know there's at least *something* you will be able to eat. We're a family of five so I feel the need to bring plenty anyway. Usually I'll take all 3 things: a protein, a vegetable (usually a salad), and a paleo treat that vanishes within seconds. That way the kids don't feel deprived when the cake they can't eat makes an appearance. If my oldest (14) decides to eat it, she is discrete about it so the younger ones don't gang up on us. If watching the kids eat canola-oil laden potato chips makes you cringe, you can make potato or Sweet Potato Chips (see the recipe on page 47) or bring potato chips cooked in coconut oil.

3. Relax if and where you can

For example, my 4 year old will spend the day vomiting and/or with diarrhea if she has even two bites of regular pizza or anything containing gluten. If she has a whole regular cupcake, she'll be thrashing on the floor for three days. I'm not even a little bit kidding. It's possible that, as her gut heals, the effects will lessen and maybe even disappear. But, for now,

I find it important to make sure she remains 100% gluten free and paleo as often as possible. My friends are often surprised to hear that the only thing I'm 100% strict about for her and myself is remaining gluten-free. At home we're pretty hardcore, but I don't feel the need to carry the hardcore-ness with me everywhere I go. Also, my 14 year old is free to make her own choices when it comes to food. They're not always choices I agree with but, other than right before and right after her major spinal surgery for scoliosis, I feel like she is at an age where she can create her own journey when it comes to food.

4. Play damage control with superfoods

If I forecast that my kids are going to get laden with some junk foods at a certain event, I try to minimize the damage by making sure my kids have super nutrient-dense meals for a couple days before and after. For example, I'll give them twice their daily dose of Fermented Cod Liver Oil for a few days. I'll also make sure to include sardines, bone broth and organ meat as often as I can.

CHAPTER 8

BEYOND THE FOOD: THE PALEO LIFESTYLE

In the paleosphere we talk a lot about food and, heck, this book is 90% all about food but I didn't want to neglect to mention that paleo is not just a diet; it is a *lifestyle*.

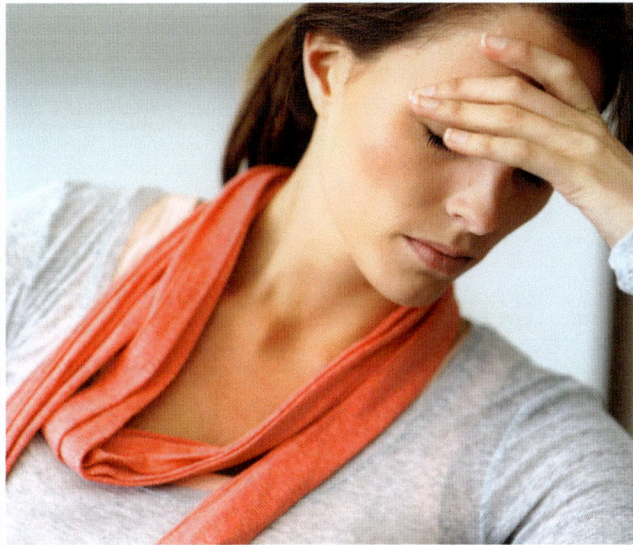

STRESS

My paleo-ish doctor once told me that diet didn't matter if I wasn't also handling my stress levels. He wasn't saying that food doesn't matter but, rather, that managing stress is just as important, if not more important, than diet. When I finally took him seriously I started experiencing even more health improvements than I did by simply adopting a paleo diet.

Acute stress is a normal function of the human body and can even be a beneficial kick in the butt to get stuff done or get the heck out of dodge. It is that "fight or flight" response we often hear about. However, stress is not meant to be chronic. In other words, the stress of a deadline which pushes us to complete a task (hello, college students) can be a good thing, and for some of us (ahem) it might be what we need in order to get things done. But experiencing this stress day in and day out from the moment you wake up till the moment you go to sleep with no end in sight is not helpful and is detrimental to our health.

Some of the common effects of stress on the body:

Stress management, adequate sleep, and exercise all contribute to our general well being just as much as proper nourishment does.

COMMON EFFECTS OF STRESS		
ON YOUR BODY	**ON YOUR MOOD**	**ON YOUR BEHAVIOR**
Headache	Anxiety	Overeating or under-eating
Muscle tension or pain	Restlessness	Angry outbursts
Chest pain	Lack of motivation or focus	Drug or alcohol abuse
Fatigue	Irritability or anger	Tobacco use
Change in sex drive	Sadness or depression	Social withdrawal
Stomach upset		
Sleep problems		

Paleo Made Easy: Getting your Family Started with the Optimal Healthy Lifestyle — with over 45 recipes!

So what can we do to manage stress?

1. Exercise

You've probably heard this one a million times but are you actually doing it? Now, I'm not talking crossfit or training for marathons. Depending on where you are in your journey, those types of exercises may actually be more of a stressor than a stress reliever. For starters, it is important to include some type of movement as this is crucial to our health and wellbeing. *Sitting is the new smoking, ya know...* For me, in times of insane work hours, I rely on my treadmill desk and fitbit to get my butt out from the chair. Is it as amazing as a hike in the woods? No, but it is a way to overcome the obstacle (read: excuse) and meet my fitness goals.

2. Meditation

This is another somewhat obvious way to address stress. When I first started meditating, I found that I couldn't go more than 30 seconds before mundane thoughts like grocery lists would make it into my head. Practice makes perfect and, while I am far from perfect, I've come a long way in my practice. Even if you begin by sitting for one minute at a time, that's a start! Try it as often as you can. I find it especially helpful to meditate before bed and before lunch. Once you make it a habit it is a lot easier to stick with it.

3. Don't sweat the small stuff

And isn't most of it small stuff? There are plenty of things that come up in life that are worth worrying about but do we really need to get our panties in a twist if a jerk cuts us off in traffic? I live in Los Angeles so believe me I have plenty of opportunities to practice my patience on this topic. It's not fair, but it's also not worth stressing about. Save arguments for things that really matter.

4. Surround yourself with people that share your goals and lifestyle

Have you noticed how your mood and disposition changes (for better or worse) after spending significant time with certain people. For instance if your boss or coworkers are negative and/or stressed out people, you're usually not skipping and singing all the way home after work. Similarly, if your friends, family, spouse or kids are happy, motivated, upbeat people, you usually go to bed with a smile on your face after a day full of laughter, friendship and collaboration. Now I know that work is work and play is play, and I know choosing your boss or coworkers is seldom easy, but I think a lot of us have much more of a say in our environment than we give ourselves cred-

it for. If your job makes you miserable, you can start to make a plan to change it. If your friends are constantly complaining about everything (I'm not talking having a bad day and needing to vent like we all sometimes do, but the ones that are constantly negative or stressed out), then get new friends. I'm serious! You don't need to "break up" with them if you don't want to, but you also don't need to subject yourself to a weekly dose of the blues. I joke that my friend "intake form" is much more rigorous now than it used to be and quality over quantity is where it's at.

5. Schedule some stress management

Now I'm not saying this to stress you out! :) That would be silly. As a wife and mother of three, I realize that if I don't schedule time for myself and simply rely on time "leftovers" for myself it just won't happen! So every 2 or 3 weeks I go see my acupuncturist. It is that easy: I just make the appointment and show up. But what about the daily meditating and getting your butt to bed on time? Well, if the scheduling works so well for the acupuncture why not schedule the meditation and sleep? That's right. I make appointments with myself. And, *doggone it,* I keep 'em! I make it a habit to meditate on my lunch break right before eating (which is super helpful for digestion) and I have an alarm on my phone for 9pm when its time to stop messing around (or blogging as it were) on the computer and start getting ready for bed with the goal of being asleep at 10pm. At first it might be tricky to make this a routine but, as you get used to it, it becomes like teeth brushing- a habit you'd have trouble skipping. Until then, schedule it!

6. Get stuff OFF your plate

If you're the typical American you're most likely racing from point A to point B, perhaps trying to be the perfect parent while also juggling a hectic career and making sure the dog gets fed. If this sounds familiar, then you can't afford NOT to get help. I don't mean hiring an entourage, (although, if that's in the budget, heck yeah go for it!) but you can stop trying to be superwoman/man. Outsource and automate what you can so you don't have to do it all. That can be anything from hiring help to joining a CSA so you're produce shows up at your doorstep or using Amazon Prime and Subscribe and Save so you're not spending two hours at the store trying to save $10. For me I had a "duh" moment this year when I finally decided to spend a few dollars on a meal plan subscription. Life changing.

7. Say NO

Yes, I'm talking about those volunteer positions at your kid's school, church, etc. This is part of the superwoman/man thing I mentioned in #6 above.

"The difference between successful people and very successful people is that very successful people say 'no' to almost everything."—Warren Buffett

Granted, he was referring to business, not stress management, but I think it can apply here as well. The bottom line (pun intended) is that, if being a superhero comes at the cost of your health or your family's well being, it's not worth it.

8. Get stuff OFF your mind!

My godfather used to tell me this as a teen (I was one wound-up teen that was over scheduled and overcommitted to a lot of things). He told me to write things down in a notebook so they're not taking up space in my head. It took me a few times of hearing this before I stopped rolling my eyes and actually tried it. It seems so simple and basic, yet it works! One of my mentors, Marie Forleo, calls it "creating mental white space". I'll take it! If you find yourself waking up in the middle of the night thinking about all the things you have to do the next day, keep a notebook by your bed and write them down. You'll be much more likely to go back to sleep without trying to remember it throughout the night and the bonus is that those things might actually get done! This, in combination with taking a few moments to write things down *before* bedtime to get ready for the next day, will be sure to take your heart rate down a few notches.

SLEEP

We all know that sleep is important, but a lot of us just don't realize *how* important (or we'd all be getting ourselves into bed instead of fiddling online throughout the night). Lack of sleep is linked to a hodgepodge of problems like obesity, high blood pressure, cardiovascular disease, inflammation, and elevated cholesterol levels. And then there are the obvious problems like crankiness and getting sick more frequently.

The scary thing is that it doesn't take much sleep deprivation to take a toll on the body. Just a night of going without sleep can mess up your metabolism, cause inflammation, and disrupt hormones[16,17].

I know we are all busy and finding time for a full 7 to 9 hours of sleep might seem impossible. Even if you do find time for sleep, you can end up tossing and turning in bed instead of getting the snooze you need. But, if you follow steps to reduce stress, like stop trying to be a superhero and sweating the small stuff, you will find that you've got plenty of time for sleep and getting to bed is a lot easier.

Unfortunately though, there is a bit of a Catch 22 here: if you don't get enough sleep, it will be harder to get rid of stress. And if you don't get rid of stress, then you will have a hard time getting enough sleep. Just do your best in each of these areas and pretty soon you'll start noticing some significant changes.

If your problem is that you aren't getting enough sleep, then consider setting a sleep curfew. Yes, get an actual alarm clock to go off and force yourself into bed at that time! If you have trouble falling asleep, then set up a go-to-sleep ritual. This can involve sipping some chamomile tea while soaking in a bath with Epsom salts and listening to some relaxing music. Ideally you would want to stay away from the computer and TV for at least an hour before bed. The blue light from these screens affects our melatonin (hormone that helps regulate sleep) production. That means your body is going to be really confused and alert instead of feeling sleepy![18] On the days that I work late on the computer or decide to watch a movie in the evening, I use special glasses that block the blue light. I also have a f.lux program on my Mac that dims according to the time of day.

Set yourself up for a successful night's sleep by limiting your caffeine intake to morning only. Some people find that they need to get rid of caffeine altogether while others are ok as long as they don't consume coffee or tea after noon. Figure out what works best for you.

Ensuring your room is completely pitch black is also essential. Use blackout curtains or a sleep mask to help you achieve the darkness you need to signal to your body and mind that it's time to rest. Earplugs and/or white noise are also very helpful. If you have kids that wake up during the night, perhaps you and your partner can take turns using earplugs so that you can achieve a solid night's sleep at least some of the time.

EXERCISE

If you read my blog, you may have noticed that I don't write about exercise often. That's because it's not my forte.

It took me a while before I started getting the exercise I need. Even as a kid, I couldn't exercise or participate in sports often because of my congenital heart condition. My mom would even call me in from playing in the snow to take frequent breaks out of fear that I would scare the crap out of her with another uncontrollable episode of tachycardia. As an adult, exercise was something I knew I should do but struggled to make a habit of. I was an expert with excuses: *I've got a health problems, I'm working two jobs, I've got 3 kids...*

These might seem like legit excuses for not exercising, but there are really no legit excuses for not exercising. If you are really motivated enough, then you can overcome any obstacle that is keeping you from exercising. And therein lies the problem: you've got to get motivated!

Ironically, the best motivation for exercising is exercise itself. It will be hard (read: frustrating, painful, exhausting...) at first. But, after just a short while, you will start feeling a lot better and noticing health benefits. These results will motivate you to keep on exercising.

Even now, several years after my heart catheter ablation that permanently "fixed" me, I'm not exactly what you would call athletic, but I understand the importance of making it a priority since **exercise is not only necessary for health; it is a keystone of mood and psychological well-being.**

Exercise triggers chemical responses in your brain, which make you feel happy. You may have heard of "runner's high" before. Well, it is from the rush of endorphins caused during exercise. The benefits can last long after your workout is over, giving you mental clarity and calmness[19]. And if you're anything like me, that will come in handy.

Exercise detoxifies your body from the inside out, boosts your brain power, improves muscle tone and skin health, improves digestion, and helps you sleep better.

How to Get Exercise into Your Busy Schedule

You don't need to follow the training schedule of an Olympic athlete to benefit from exercise. Any movement is better than none! At the moment, I take a yoga class at least once a week and work on my treadmill desk from Monday to Friday. I aim for 70,000 steps per week, which I track with my fitbit. I also fit in kettlebell workouts from home 3 times per week, which I love because it only takes 15–20 minutes to really get.it.done. Efficiency is my middle name! Hikes on the weekend with the family a couple times a month are also one of my favorite things to do.

When you are just starting out and dealing with many changes, you may want to stick to gentle forms of exercise. Don't try to be a hero and push yourself too hard; you might just end up getting burnt out. One of my favorite gentle exercises is gardening. It is very physical, but can be done at your own pace. I also find it relaxing and, as a bonus, gardening helps me feed my family while also keeping me in shape.

If you are a parent, then you've probably noticed that kids are never still for very long. They're running from one place to the next, squatting to pick something up and toss it, etc. No wonder they're in such great shape! One of the best ways to get exercise is simply to play with your kids. If your kids are anything like mine, they are overjoyed when you stop everything to spend some time playing with them. It doesn't have to be an organized game and you don't need to pull out the clown costume. Just play. You can play tag, hide and seek, pretend you are various creatures crawling around, build sand castles, or just get on the playground equipment and be silly. The bonus? It makes such a difference in stress levels of both parent and child, and connects you to your kids on a whole different level.

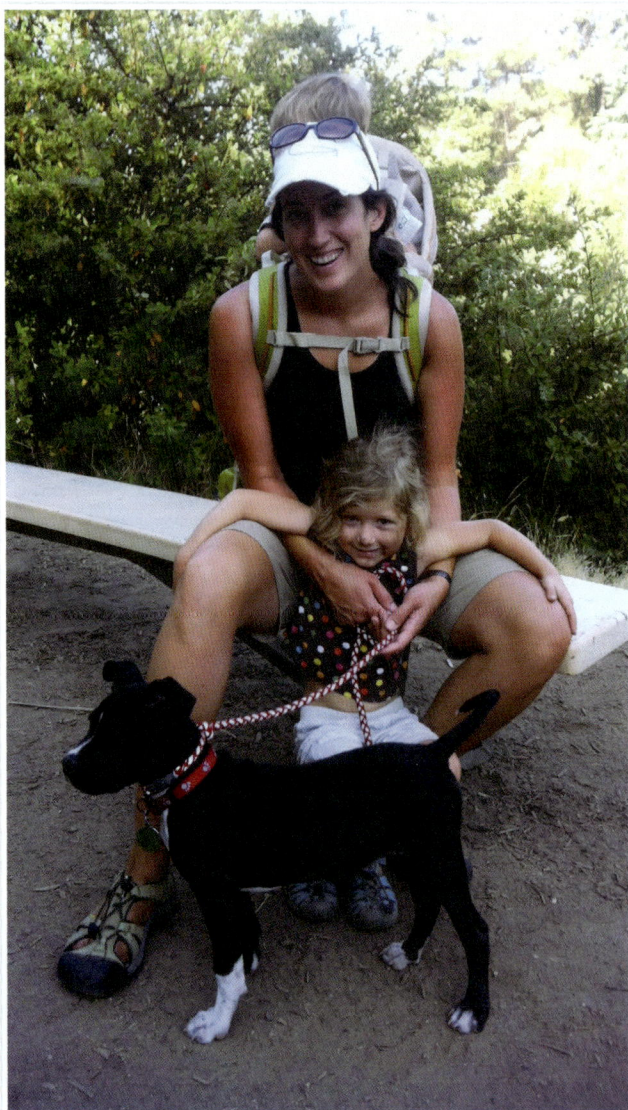

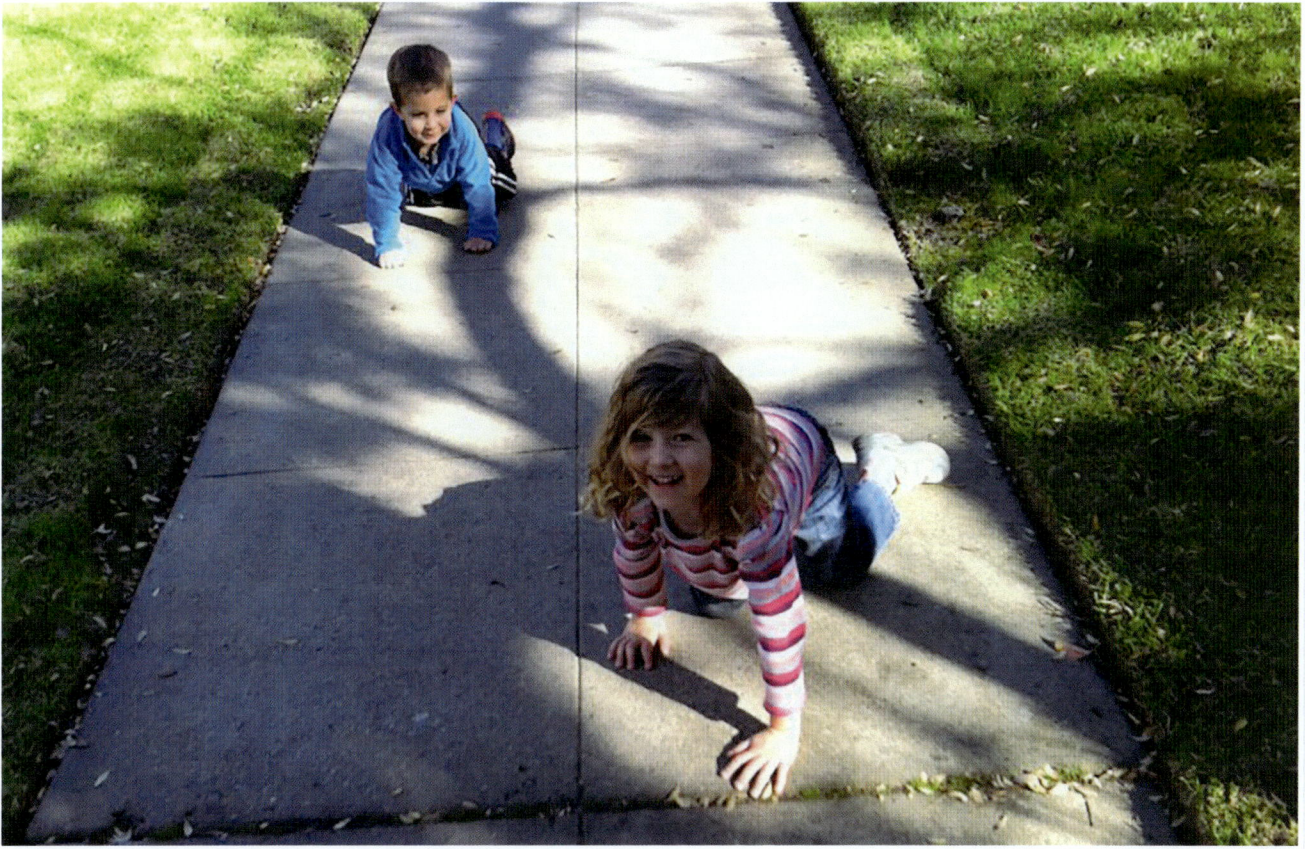

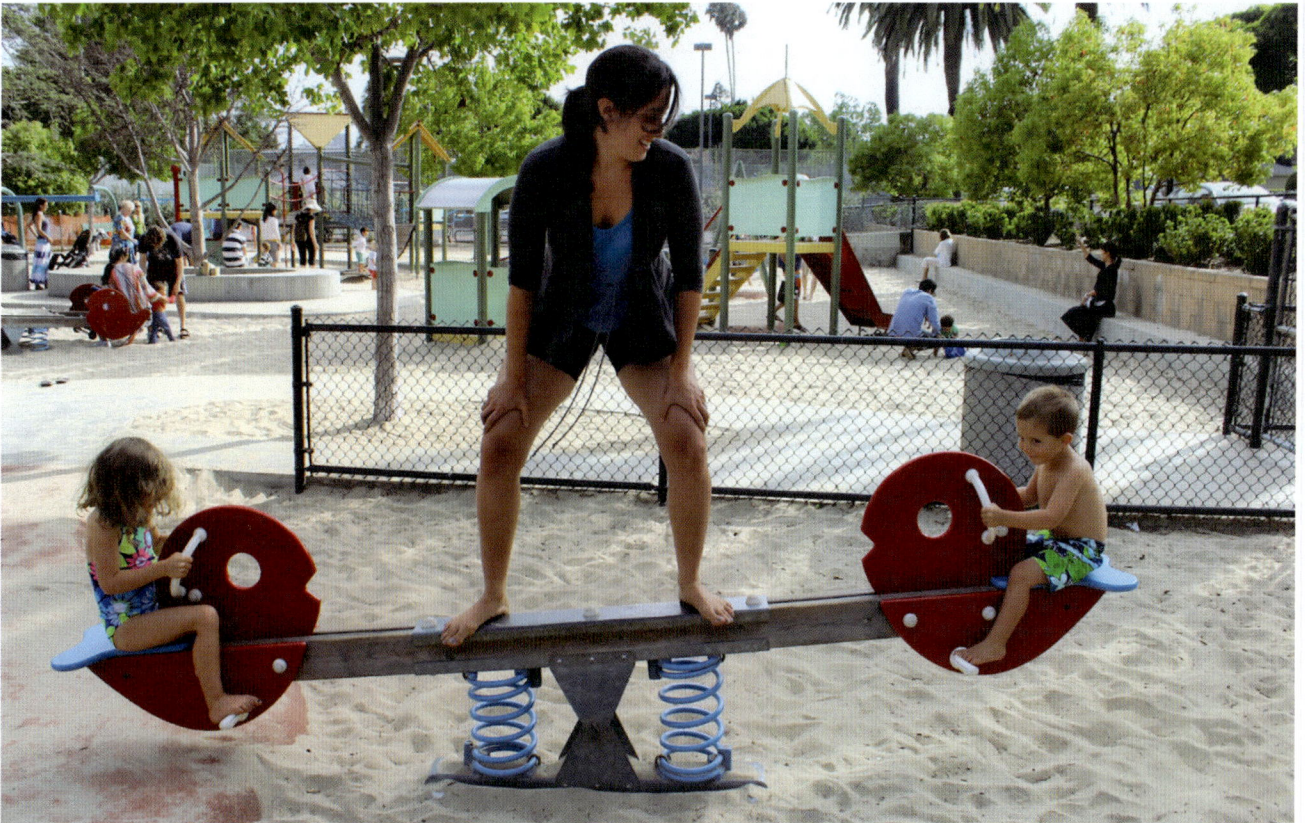

Paleo Made Easy: Getting your Family Started with the Optimal Healthy Lifestyle—with over 45 recipes!

MEAT

CHIMICHURRI MEATBALLS

Chimichurri is a sauce usually used for grilled meat in Argentina where I grew up.
Here is a simple way to replicate that favor and spice up meatballs!

Ingredients:

¼ cup (approx) of chopped fresh parsley | 2 garlic cloves, minced | 1½ tsp. sea salt

½ tsp of pepper | 2 lbs grass-fed ground beef

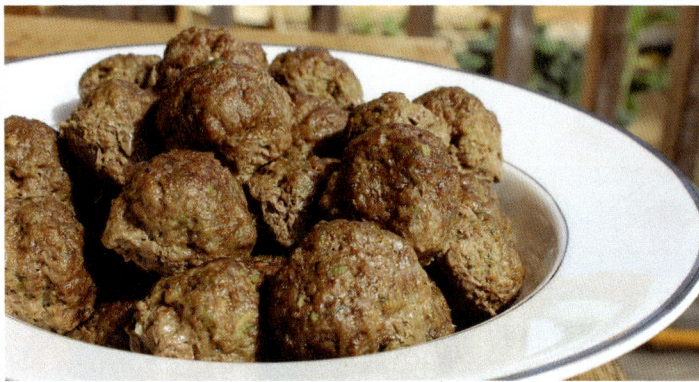

Directions:

1. In a large bowl combine the chopped parsley, minced garlic, sea salt, pepper and ground beef.

2. Mix well.

3. Roll into medium size meatballs (approx 20–25).

4. Place into a baking pan or dish.

5. Bake for 30–40 minutes at 350 degrees.

6. Enjoy!

CRISPY FISH NUGGETS

What you will need:

3 cups palm or coconut oil | 2 cans wild caught tuna | 2 cans wild caught salmon

2 cans wild caught sardines | ½ cup and 2 Tbsp. arrowroot powder | 2 eggs

1 tsp. sea salt | 1 tsp. pepper

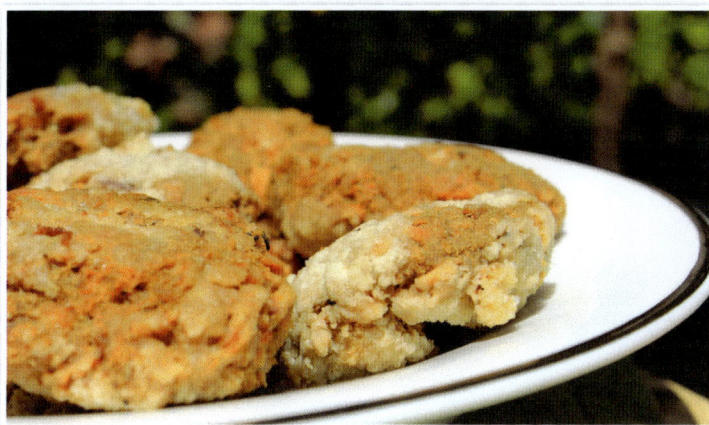

Directions:

1. Heat oil in a deep sided pan on high.

2. In a bowl mix together the fish, eggs and 2 Tbsp. arrowroot powder.

3. On a separate dish mix ½ cup arrowroot powder with 1 tsp. salt and 1 tsp. pepper.

4. Shape fish and coat it with the arrowroot mixture.

5. Place in oil and cook nuggets until golden brown.

6. Remove and enjoy!

Paleo Made Easy: Getting your Family Started with the Optimal Healthy Lifestyle—with over 45 recipes!

CINNAMON SLIDERS

We eat a lot of ground beef around here... It is inexpensive and versatile and great for last minute dinner prep. The trick to not getting bored with it is to change up the spices! Here is a super simple recipe:

What you will need:

2 lbs ground beef | 2 tsp. cinnamon | 1 tsp. sea salt

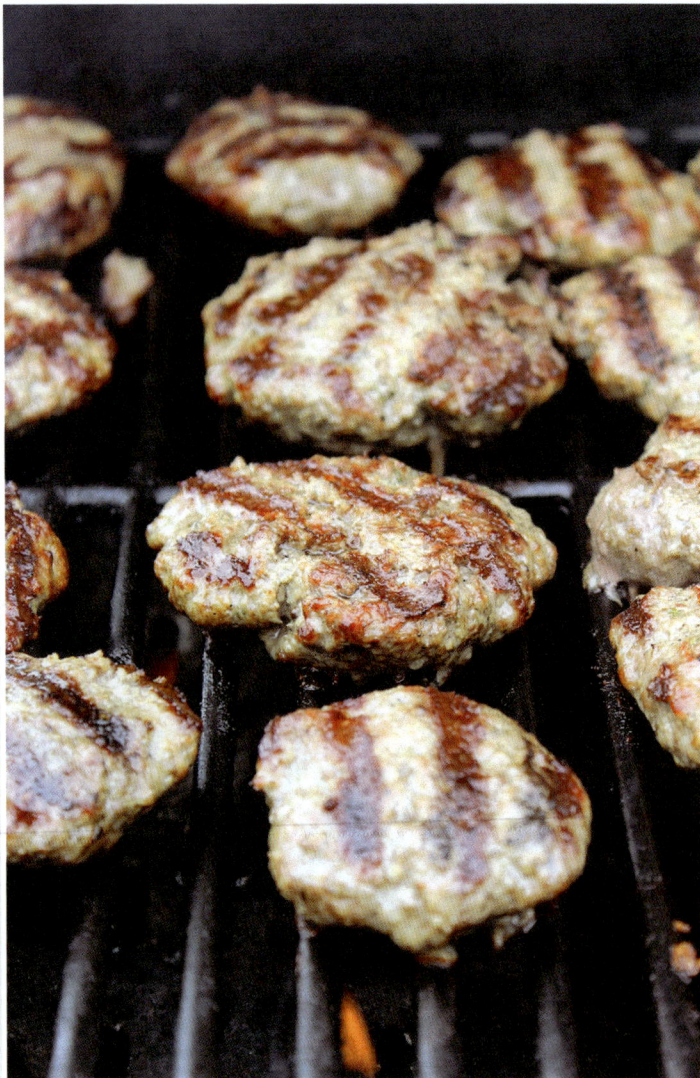

Directions

1. Mix all ingredients well.

2. Shape into small patties.

3. BBQ for 5–10 minutes on each side at 350–400 degrees.

4. Enjoy!

Paleo Made Easy: Getting your Family Started with the Optional Healthy Lifestyle—with over 45 recipes!

3-MINUTE STEAK RUB

What you will need:

1 tsp salt | ½ tsp organic garlic powder | ¼ teaspoon organic cinnamon

¼ tsp organic cumin powder | 1.5 lb skirt or flank steak

Directions:

1. Mix the spices well.

2. Rub evenly on both sides of the steak.

3. Throw it on the grill and cook until the steak reaches at least 140 degrees.

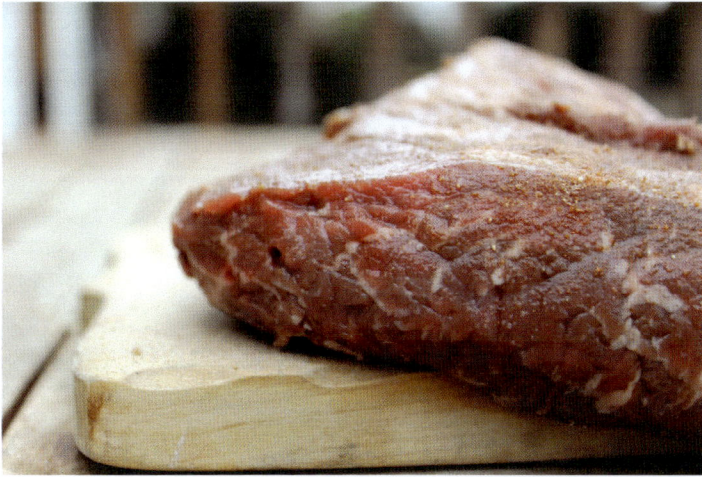

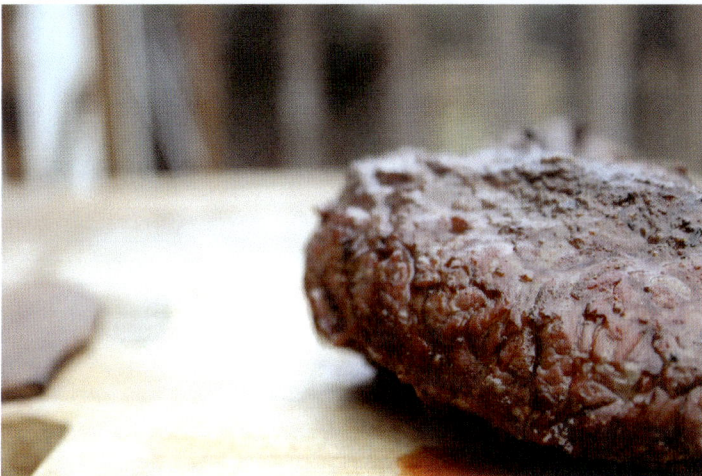

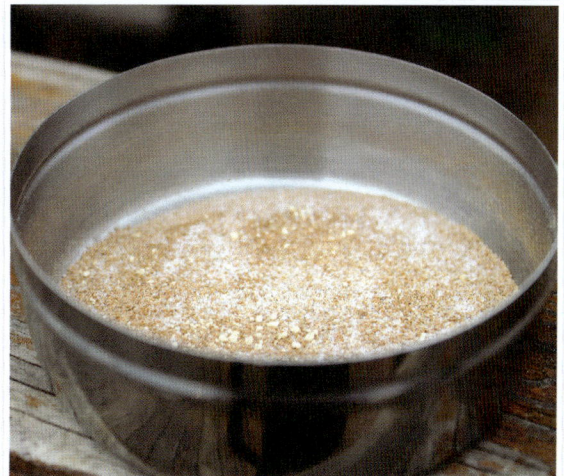

4. SO GOOD!

Paleo Made Easy: Getting your Family Started with the Optimal Healthy Lifestyle—with over 45 recipes!

EASY-PEASY SLOW COOKER CHICKEN

What you will need:

A slow cooker | 2 small chickens or 1 large one (preferably pastured) | 1 small bunch of fresh rosemary

1 Tbsp. salt | 1 tsp. pepper | 2 onions | 2 carrots, optional

2 cloves of garlic | 2 Tbsp. grass-fed ghee

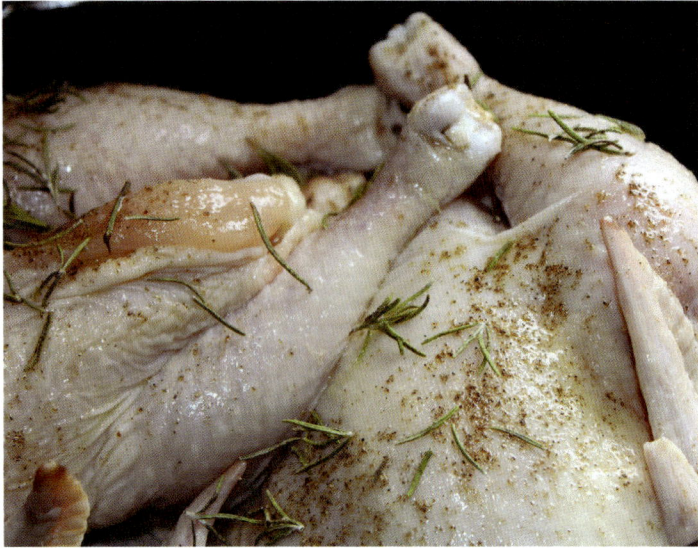

Directions:

1. Roughly chop onion, carrots and garlic and add to the slow cooker

2. Place chicken on top of chopped vegetables

3. Drip the ghee over the chicken.

4. Add salt, pepper and rosemary.

5. Cover and let cook on medium for 6–8 hours or until 170 degrees.

6. Serve with our Mashed Cauliflower on page 48 for a yummy comfort meal.

7. Enjoy!

Paleo Made Easy: Getting your Family Started
with the Optimal Healthy Lifestyle—with over 45 recipes!

HIDDEN LIVER BURGERS

Grass-fed liver is an excellent source of vitamins A, D and K2. It is one of the best superfoods you can eat!
The thing is, unless you were raised eating organ meats, chances are it is not gonna be your favorite.
No worries—just sneak it in!

What you will need:

4 lbs. grass-fed ground beef | 1 Tbsp. sea salt | 2 Tbsp. dried sage | 1 Tbsp. onion powder

4 Tbsp. (approx.) of grass fed liver—add more if you're brave!

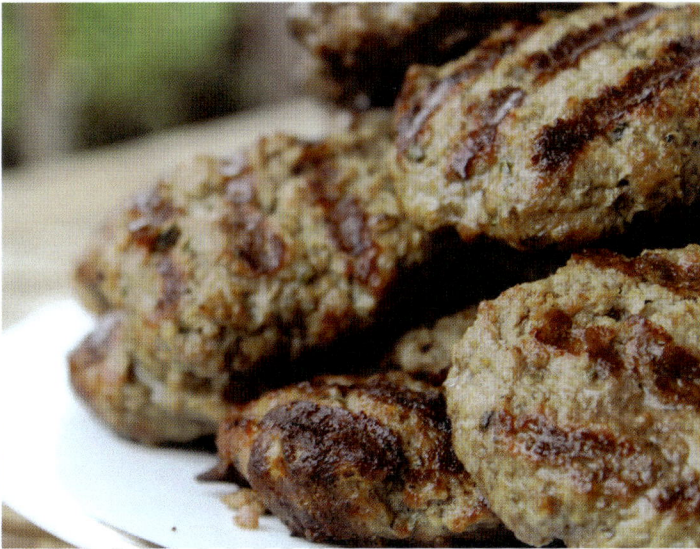

Directions:

1. Grind liver in food processor
2. Combine all ingredients
3. Shape into patties and put them on the BBQ (350–400 degrees).
4. Cook for 5–10 minutes on each side.
5. Enjoy!

PULLED PORK

When we have a long day outside the house, our slow cooker becomes a lifesaver!

What you will need:

A slow cooker | 4–5 lb pork shoulder roast, preferably pastured | 1 large onion

3 cloves of garlic | ¼ cup yellow mustard | ¼ cup maple syrup | ½ tsp. all-spice

1 Tbsp. salt | 1 cup pureed tomato | Cream from the top of one can (13.5 oz) of coconut milk

½ cup beef or chicken broth, preferably homemade

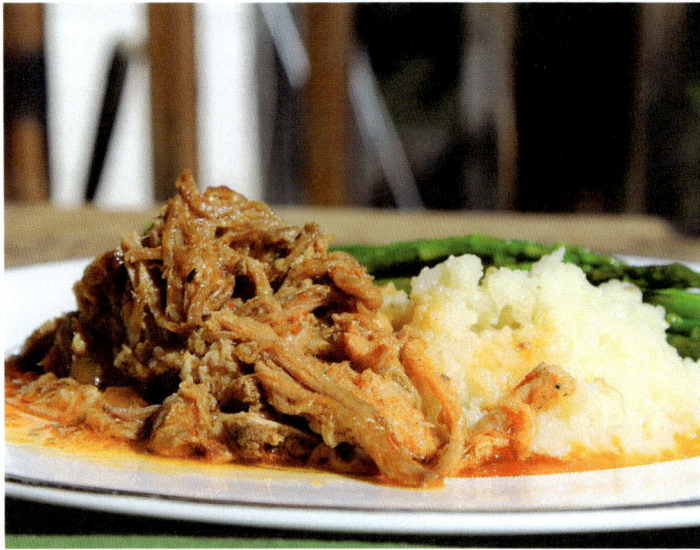

Directions:

1. Dice onion and mince garlic.

2. Mix all ingredients except the roast and place in the slow cooker on low.

3. Use a skillet to sear the roast on all sides on medium high heat.

4. Place the roast in the slow cooker and cook on low for 6–8 hours.

5. After 6 hours or so, shred the pork with a fork (it should shred easily) and mix with the sauce that has formed in the slow cooker.

6. Serve and enjoy!

Paleo Made Easy: Getting your Family Started with the Optimal Healthy Lifestyle—with over 45 recipes!

SIDE DISHES

CRISPY SWEET POTATO CHIPS

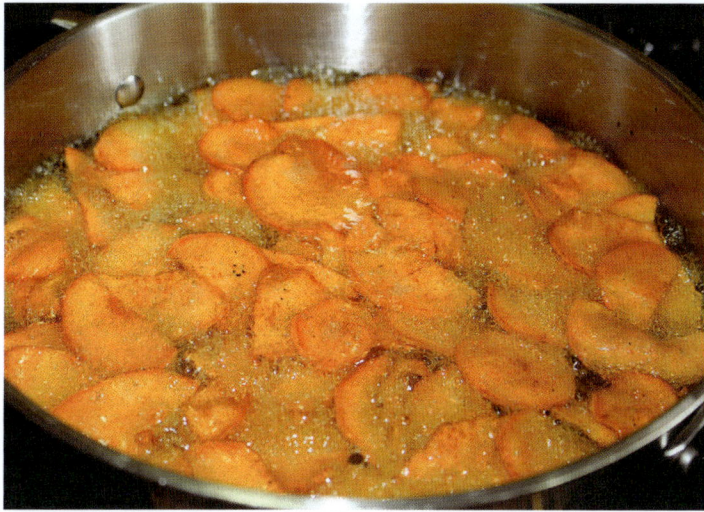

Directions:

1. Peel sweet potatoes.

2. Slice thinly (I like to use the slicing tool on my food processor).

3. Salt and pepper the slices before frying—this is key!

4. Fry in coconut oil until brown (you can strain and save the oil to use up to 12 times)

5. Set on paper towels to soak up the grease

6. Enjoy! (or: break up fights between the kids that are hogging them)

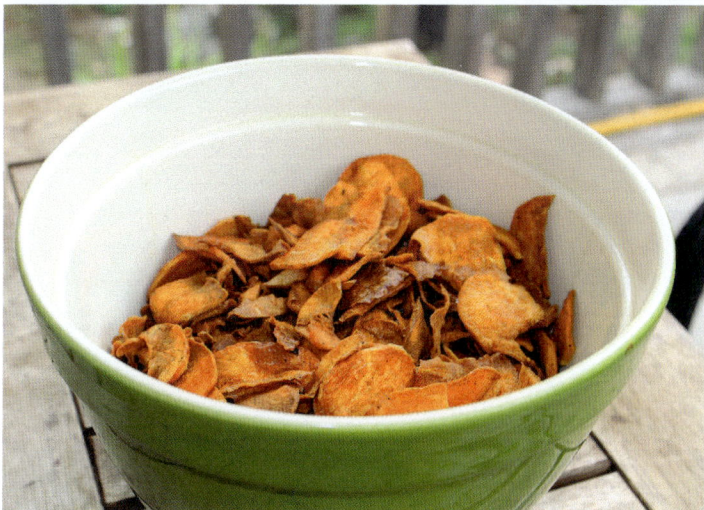

ORGANIC KALE CHIPS

What you will need:

2 bunches of kale | ½ cup coconut oil | sea salt to taste

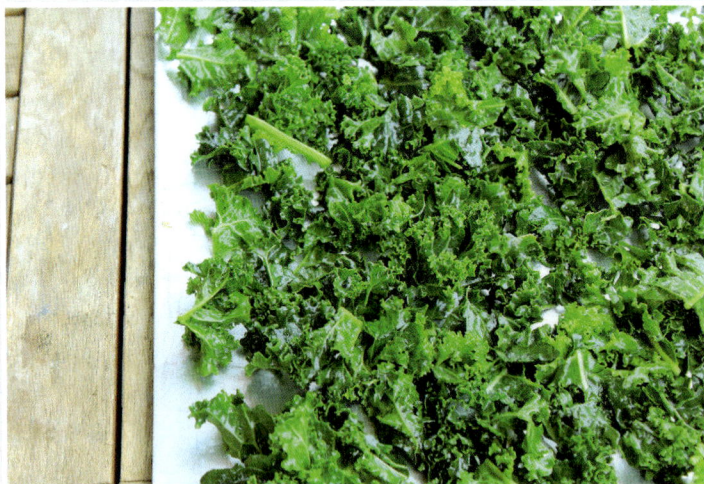

Directions:

1. Wash and dry kale and remove leaves from the stem.
2. Place in bowl and add salt and oil.
3. Mix well and place on a baking sheet.
4. Bake for 30 minutes at 250 degrees.
5. Enjoy!

MASHED CAULIFLOWER

These are a great side dish to any meat when you want some filling comfort food.

What you will need:

2 heads of cauliflower | Grass-fed ghee | Salt | Pepper

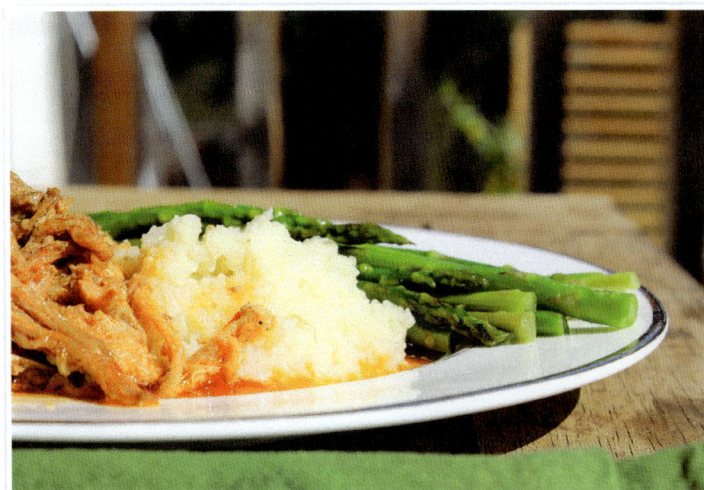

Directions:

1. Wash and cut cauliflower.
2. Steam the cauliflower for 15–20 minutes (it should be easy to pierce with a fork)
3. Mash in a pot with ghee.
4. Add salt and pepper to taste.
5. Enjoy!

Paleo Made Easy: Getting your Family Started with the Optimal Healthy Lifestyle—with over 45 recipes!

SWEET POTATOES WITH PECAN CRUST

For the Sweet Potatoes:

4 cups mashed sweet potatoes | 2 eggs | ½ tsp. sea salt | 4 Tbsp. ghee | 1 tsp. vanilla

For the Crust:

½ cup apples, chopped | 3 Tbsp. ghee | ½ cup chopped pecans | 1 tsp cinnamon | 1 tsp vanilla

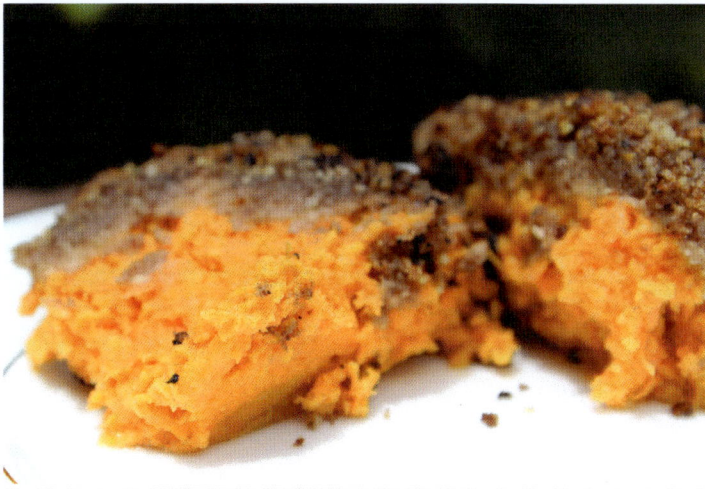

Directions:

1. Mix the sweet potatoes, eggs, 4Tbsp of ghee and vanilla and flatten onto a baking dish.

2. Put all the crust ingredients in a food processor or blender. Stop when it looks like dough.

3. Spread the crust mixture over the top of the sweet potato filling.

4. Bake for 30 minutes at 325 degrees.

5. Enjoy hot or cold!

*Paleo Made Easy: Getting your Family Started
with the Optimal Healthy Lifestyle—with over 45 recipes!*

PALEO BROCCOLI TEMPURA

I love Japanese food and I miss tempura! Traditionally, tempura is made with wheat flour
and fried in god-knows-what. Luckily there's a paleo version you can enjoy!

What you will need:

1.5 cups of coconut oil or ethically sourced palm oil | Florets from 2 heads of broccoli

1 cup of almond flour | 2 eggs | ½ cup coconut milk | 1 tsp. sea salt

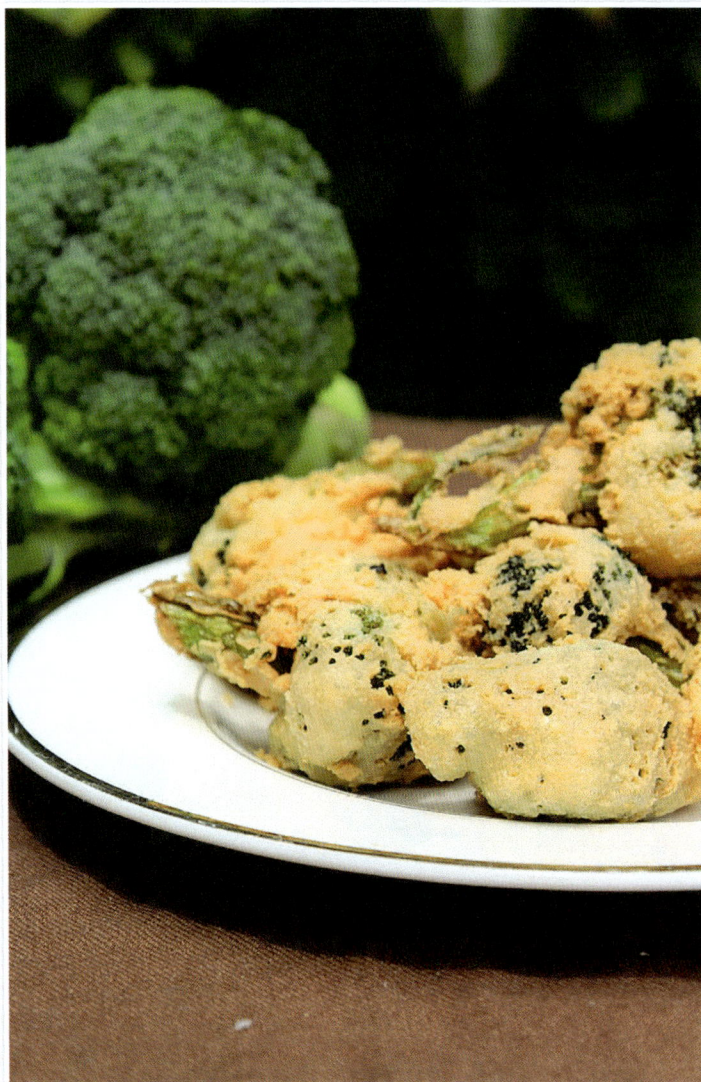

Directions:

1. Put oil in a deep pan and turn on high.

2. Put all ingredients (excluding broccoli) in a food processor or blender.

3. Mix until it looks like batter.

4. Dip your broccoli in the batter and carefully place in the hot oil.

5. Use tongs to turn broccoli until it is light brown on all sides.

6. Remove from oil and let cool.

7. Enjoy!

*Paleo Made Easy: Getting your Family Started
with the Optimal Healthy Lifestyle—with over 45 recipes!*

SUPER EASY CAULIFLOWER RICE

What you will need:

Food processor | 1 large head of cauliflower

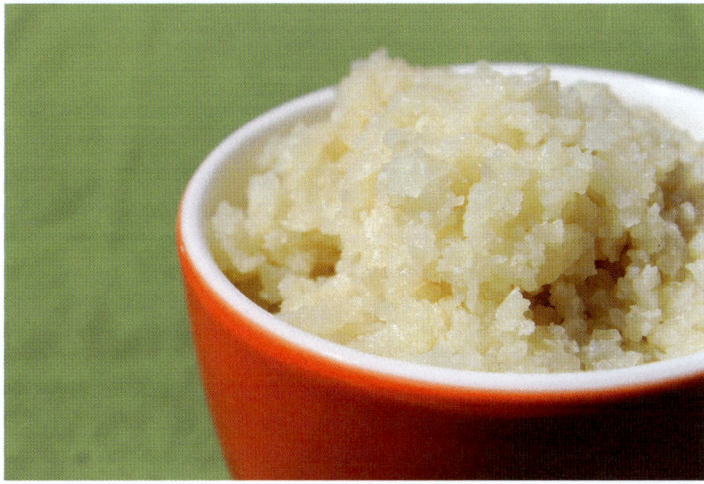

Directions:

1. Chop cauliflower until it resembles rice.

2. Put in a pot on low heat.

3. Mix occasionally until hot.

4. Turn off heat and let sit

5. Enjoy with your favorite sauce or simply topped with butter or ghee!

Paleo Made Easy: Getting your Family Started with the Optimal Healthy Lifestyle—with over 45 recipes!

SALT AND PEPPER SWEET POTATO FRIES

Did you know that sweet potato fries at restaurants are often floured? For those of us that try so hard to remain 100% gluten free, that can be a big disappointment! Of course there's also the issue of rancid seed oils they're usually fried in as well. The reason they're floured is because that's the only way to get them crispy. If you want to replicate the crispy sweet potato fries you love but fry them in healthy, delicious saturated fat and keep them 100% gluten free, this is the recipe for you!

Yup, these are just as delicious as they look :)

What you will need:

3 large sweet potatoes | 4 cups of palm or coconut oil | 2 eggs | ¼ cup arrowroot powder

1 tsp. sea salt | ½ tsp. pepper

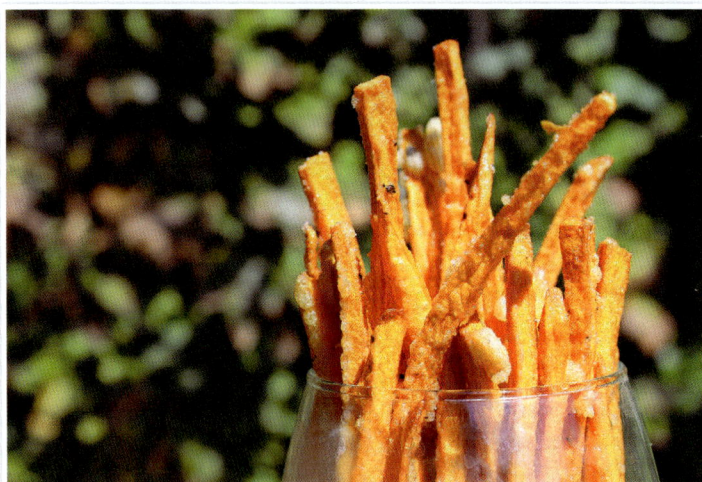

Directions:

1. Cut sweet potatoes into thin strips.

2. Heat oil in a deep pan on high heat.

3. Mix the egg, arrowroot powder, salt and pepper.

4. Lightly coat a small batch of sweet potato strips in the batter and drop into the hot oil.

5. Use tongs to move the fries around a bit to prevent sticking.

6. When golden orange, remove from the oil and place on a paper towel.

7. Repeat as necessary.

8. Season, serve and enjoy!

9. You can re-use the frying oil as many as 12 times, so save it for next time!

Paleo Made Easy: Getting your Family Started with the Optimal Healthy Lifestyle—with over 45 recipes!

SALADS

PALEO TACO SALAD (Minus the Taco)

This is one of our family's favorites! If you just can't fathom having it without the crunch, add some chopped jicama!

What you will need:

2 pounds of grass-fed ground beef | 1 lb. cooked pastured bacon ends and pieces for bacon bits

1 large head of lettuce | 2 tomatoes | 3 small avocados or 2 large

2 apples, or other fruit of your choice | ¼ cup extra virgin olive oil | ¼ cup organic apple cider vinegar

salt and pepper to taste | Chimichurri Sauce (optional) recipe on page 74

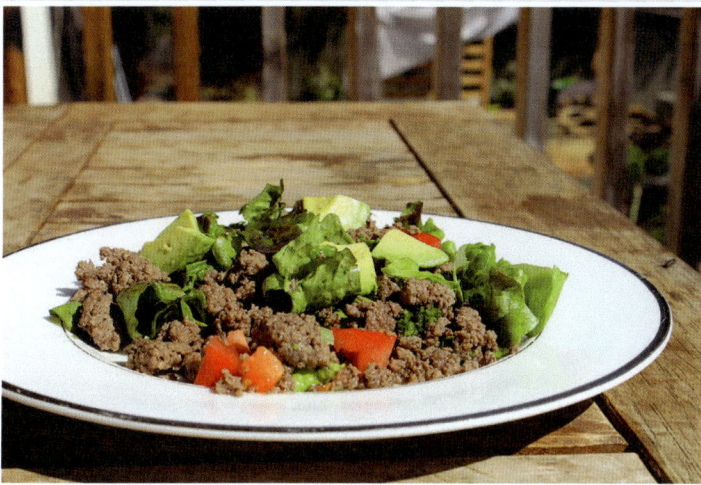

Directions:

1. Fry the ground beef and flavor with salt and pepper.

2. Mix the salad with the vinegar, oil, salt and a little pepper.

3. Sprinkle some chopped apples on top.

4. Add the chopped tomato and avocado.

5. Add some chimichurri.

6. Add some ground beef.

7. Add some bacon bits.

8. Enjoy!

The great thing about this recipe is that most of it can be prepared ahead of time. I wash and chop the tomatoes, fruit and lettuce earlier in the day and keep them in the fridge. That leaves cutting up some avocado and cooking the ground beef. The quantities above are really just a starting point and the recipe often becomes a "what's in the fridge" salad.

SWEET AND SOUR KALE SALAD

We have a lot of kale in our garden. Here is one of our favorite ways to use it up.

What you will need:

1 bunch of Kale	2 nectarines	¼ lb. of dried cranberries	¼ lb. pine nuts
¼ cup extra virgin olive oil	¼ cup organic apple cider vinegar	salt and pepper to taste	

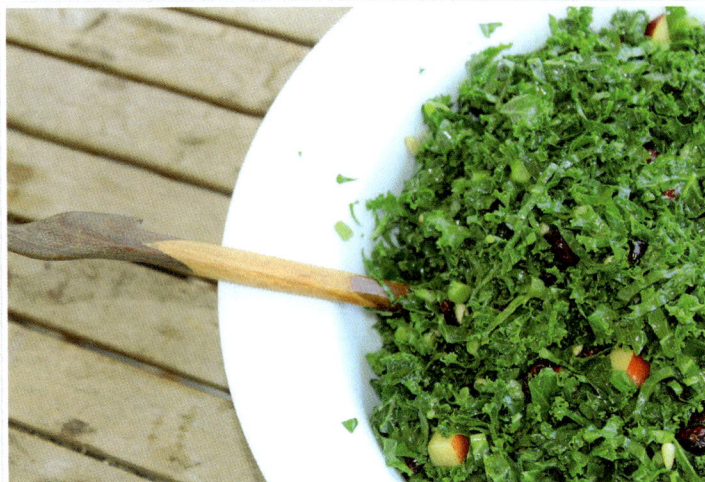

Directions:

1. The key to any kale salad is to chop it as finely as possible, so spend some time chopping.

2. Cut the nectarines into small chunks.

3. Add the pine nuts and dried cranberries.

4. Add the olive oil and vinegar.

5. Add salt and pepper to taste.

6. Toss and enjoy!

The great thing about kale is that it holds up a lot longer than lettuce once it's dressed, so even if you make the salad well before dinner, it won't be soggy... still delicious!

Paleo Made Easy: Getting your Family Started with the Optimal Healthy Lifestyle—with over 45 recipes!

SIMPLE MIXED GREENS SALAD

We love the fresh kale from our garden, but sometimes we need to mix it up a bit!
So, we use a variety of greens for this salad plus some mint to make the flavors more interesting!

Ingredients:

½ bunch kale	1 bunch spinach	1 small head of red leaf lettuce	15–20 leaves of fresh mint
2 medium tomatoes	½ large lemon, juiced	¼ cup extra virgin olive oil	Salt and Pepper to taste

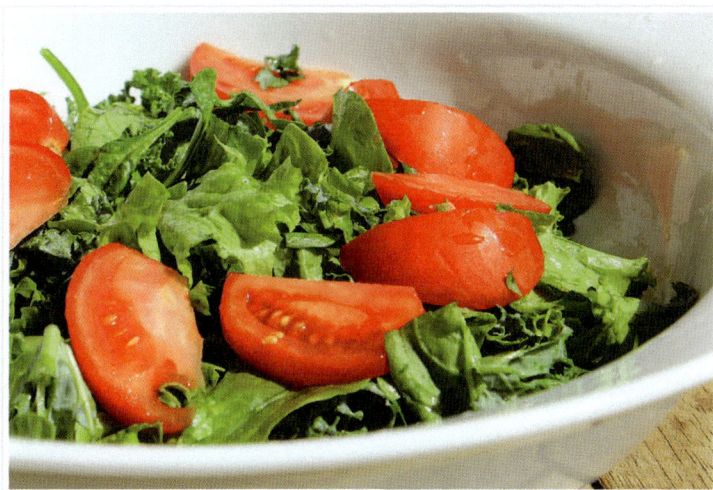

Directions:

1. Wash and chop the kale, spinach and lettuce. The kale should be very finely chopped but other greens can be in larger pieces.

2. Slice the tomatoes.

3. Put everything in a bowl and add the lemon juice, EVOO, salt and pepper.

4. Mix and enjoy!

Paleo Made Easy: Getting your Family Started with the Optimal Healthy Lifestyle—with over 45 recipes!

AVOCADO TOMATO TUNA SALAD

This is one of those "throw a bunch of things together" salads that tastes fancier than it is!
It is a really great one to take to work. I keep a 6-pack of tuna and olive oil, vinegar, salt and pepper at work
so I can just bring the produce each day in a glass jar. I toss it all together at lunchtime and lunch is served!

What you will need:

1 large head of lettuce (we like red leaf) | 2 avocados | 2 tomatoes | 2 cans of wild planet tuna

3 Tbsp. Extra Virgin Olive Oil | 3 Tbsp. Apple Cider Vinegar | Sea salt and pepper to taste

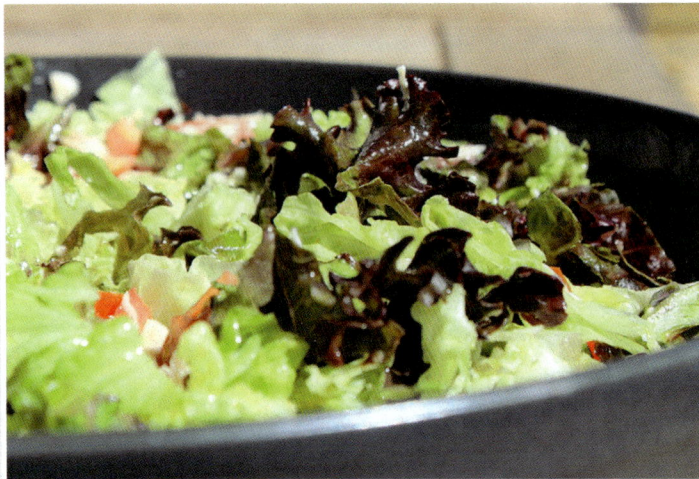

Directions:

1. Wash and chop lettuce.
2. Break up the tuna with a fork and add it to the lettuce.
3. Chop and add tomatoes and avocados.
4. Add olive oil and apple cider vinegar.
5. Add salt and pepper.
6. Toss and enjoy!

*Paleo Made Easy: Getting your Family Started
with the Optimal Healthy Lifestyle—with over 45 recipes!*

BABY BROCCOLI SALAD

What you will need:

2 heads of fresh baby broccoli | 1 small red onion | ½ pound cooked and crumbled bacon, preferably pastured

¾ cup Homemade Baconnaise (recipe on page 69) | ½ cup raisins | ½ cup pecans

¼ cup maple syrup | 2 Tbsp. apple cider vinegar

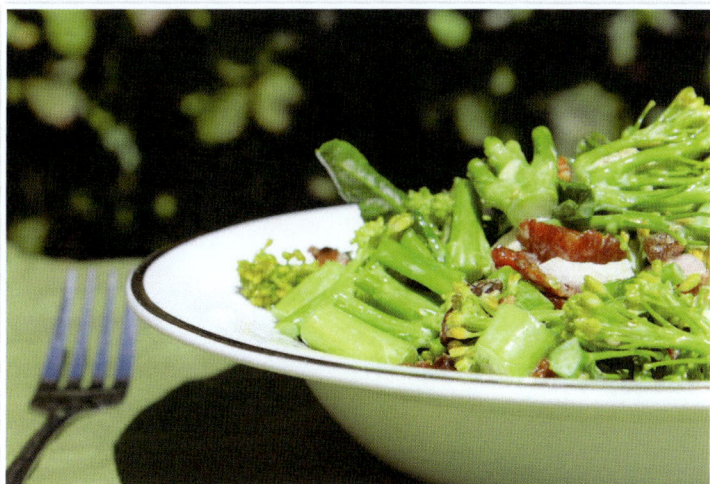

Directions:

1. Cook and crumble your bacon.
2. Cut the broccoli into bite size pieces.
3. Chop the onion finely
4. Combine all ingredients in bowl and mix well.
5. Chill and serve.
6. Enjoy!

Paleo Made Easy: Getting your Family Started
with the Optimal Healthy Lifestyle — with over 45 recipes!

FERMENTED FOODS
AND BEVERAGES

HOMEMADE KOMBUCHA

Kombucha is a fermented sweet tea. It is a probiotic (contains good bacteria) and is said to help in digestion and detoxification of the body. Kombucha can often be purchased at your local health foods store but is often pricey and can be made easily at home for just a few pennies.

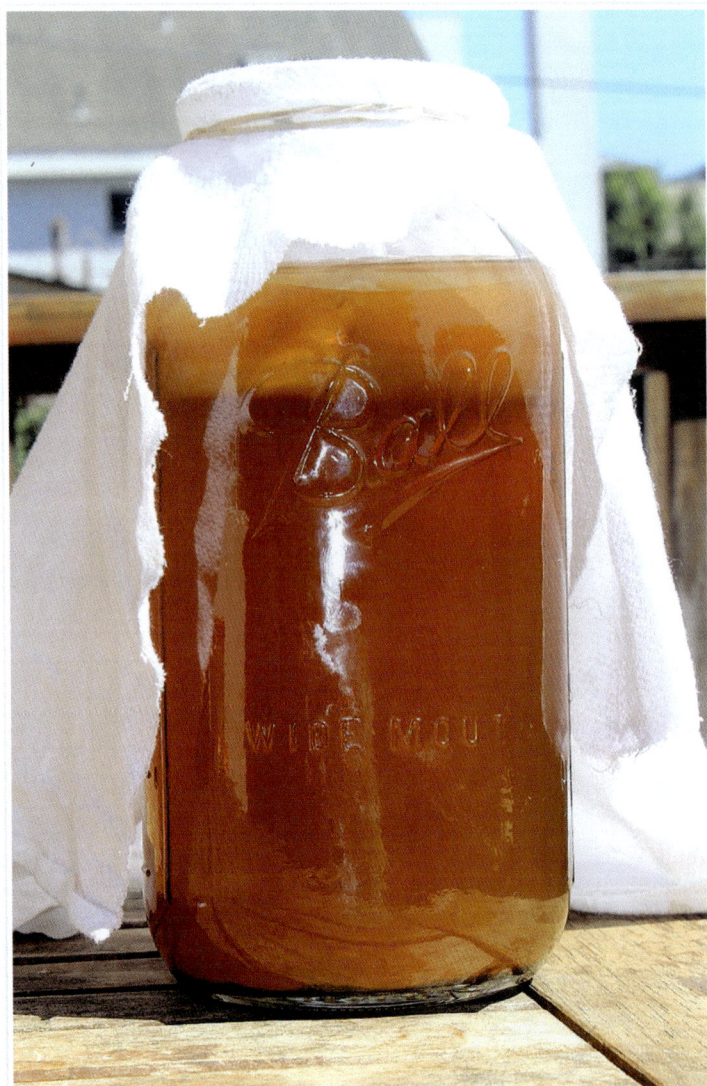

You can play around with flavoring your kombucha with several fruits. Our kids think it's soda and I love that they're drinking a gut-healthy probiotic instead.

Is it caffeinated? Is it alcoholic?

Not really. Some people say they feel the effect of a bit of a caffeine kick, others say they feel a bit of a buzz. It depends on how long you're fermenting it. The "mother" (the SCOBY) needs caffeine and sugar to grow and stay alive but the amount that remains is nominal.

HOW TO: BREW KOMBUCHA

You will need:

1 SCOBY (Symbiotic Culture Of Bacteria and Yeast) | ½ gallon mason jar or continuous brewer

1 old piece of breathable cloth (from an old tee-shirt is ideal) | 1 rubber band

4 tea bags or 2 Tbsp. of organic green or black tea (has to be caffeinated) | ½ cup organic sugar

1 large glass bowl for brewing tea

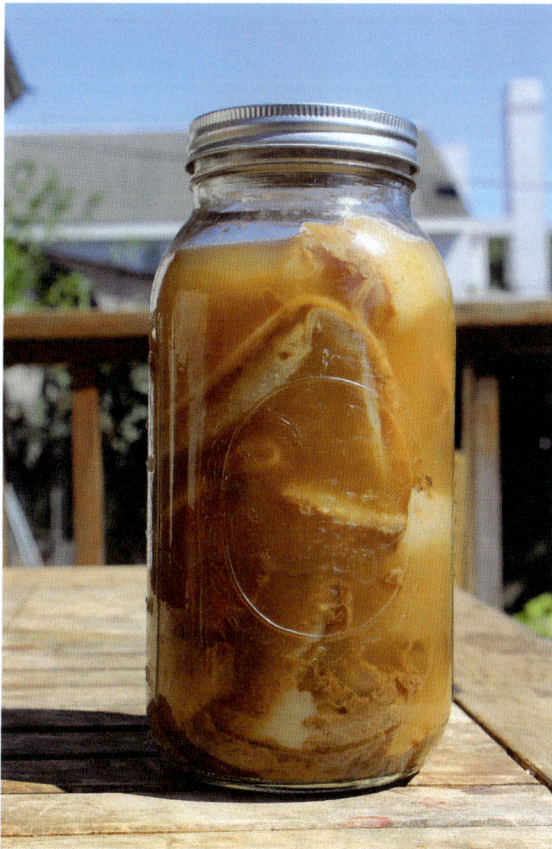

First fermentation:

1. Boil ½ gallon of water.

2. Pour ½ cup sugar into bowl.

3. Place tea bags or tea strainer with 2Tbsp loose leaf tea in center of bowl.

4. Pour boiling water over tea and sugar.

5. Dissolve sugar and let steep.

6. Place SCOBY and starter liquid in the mason jar.

7. Wait for tea to cool to room temperature—this is KEY!

8. Once cool, pour tea into jar with the SCOBY.

9. Cover the jar with cloth using the rubber band to secure it (fruit flies love this stuff so don't use cheesecloth—t-shirt material which has a tighter weave is much better)

10. Depending on the temperature and the size of the scoby the kombucha should be ready in about a week. Keep testing it until it tastes like you want it!

11. When it's ready you can bottle it in glass bottles or smaller glass jars and move on to the second fermentation.

Save that SCOBY—It will last a long time, and another one will form. Take the new one out of the jar and put it in another jar so you can start another ½ gallon. Once you have several, you can start a SCOBY hotel! Just place them all in a jar making sure the liquid is covering them. If you seal the jar with a regular lid instead of the t-shirt it will slow down the evaporation and fermentation, which is what you want for your hotel.

You can also use a continuous brewer to make larger more frequent batches with less fuss. If you're just starting out, try it with a mason jar first and move on to a continuous brewer when you're ready!

Second fermentation:

Once you bottle the kombucha after the first fermentation you can simply let it ferment as is in the bottles for a few more days and enjoy or you can flavor it at this time.

HOW TO MAKE APRICOT KOMBUCHA

We have tons of apricots on our trees, which we usually dehydrate. But they also go great in Kombucha!

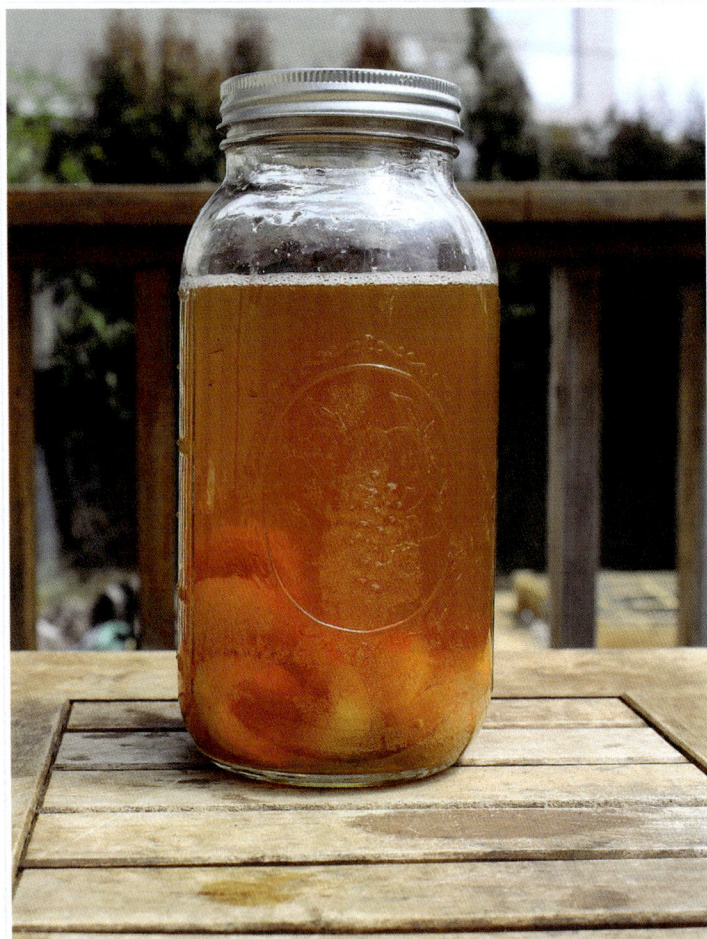

Kombucha should be flavored during the second fermentation. To flavor it with apricots, you simply:

1. Pour your fermented kombucha into a storage container with a lid.

2. Wash apricots and cut in half to remove pits.

3. Add about 5 apricots to your kombucha.

4. Replace the lid and wait 5–7 days to infuse the apricot flavor.

5. Enjoy! (if you can beat the kids to it).

6. You can either strain the apricots out and toss them in the compost bin or eat them if you dare!

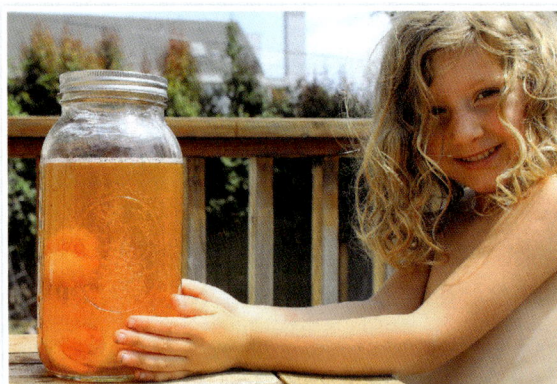

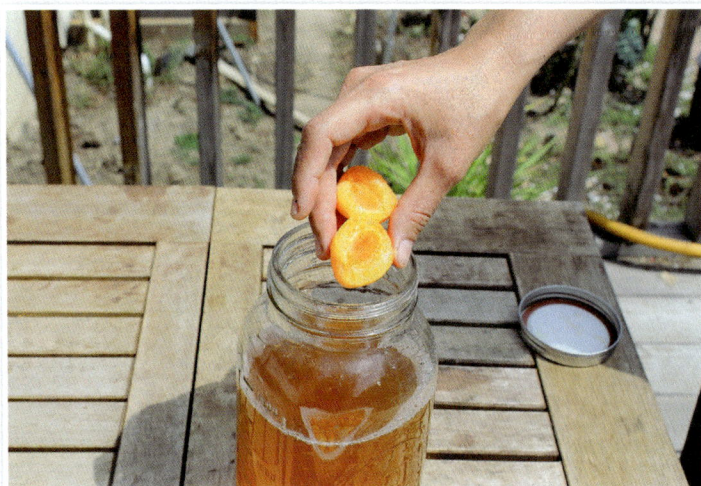

Paleo Made Easy: Getting your Family Started with the Optimal Healthy Lifestyle—with over 45 recipes!

STRAWBERRY KOMBUCHA

When we buy strawberries at the farmers market, the biggest, juiciest ones are always on top. By the time we make our way to the bottom of the basket, they get a little bruised. So what do you do with the bruised berries at the bottom of the basket? Because we pretty much have a kombucha factory in our kitchen, we use them to flavor our kombucha!

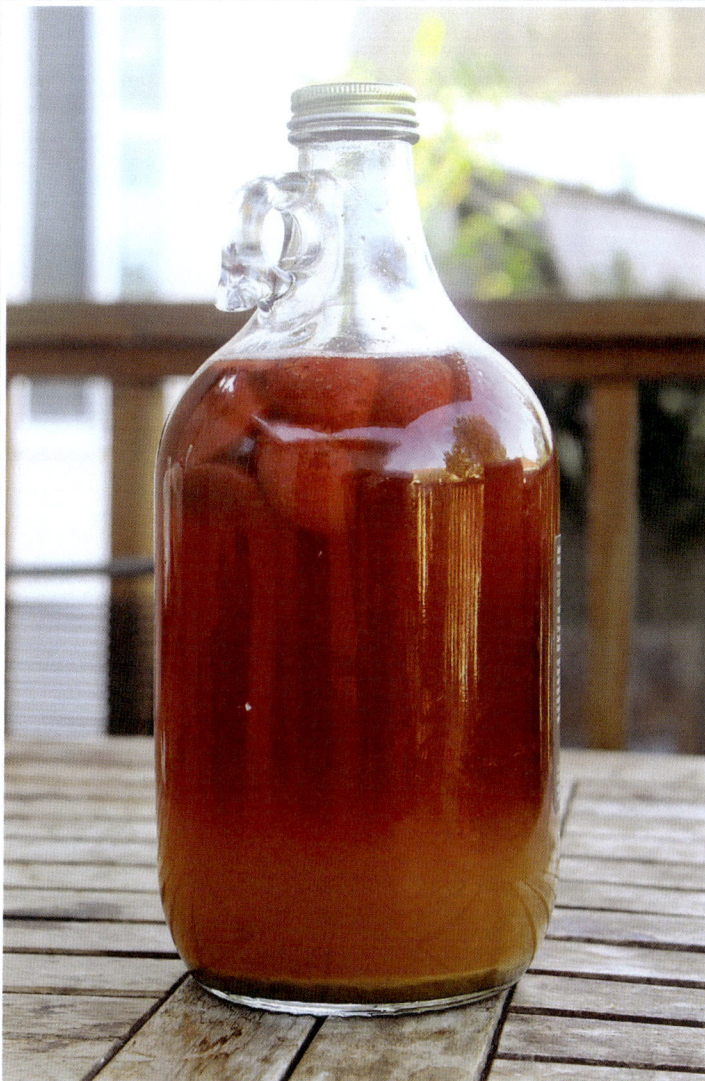

After the initial fermenting process we separate our "good" strawberries from the bruised ones.

The berries we don't want to eat go directly into the kombucha bottle during the secondary fermentation, which both flavors and carbonates the kombucha. The kombucha sucks the flavor and color from the strawberries pretty quickly, and a few days later you have strawberry kombucha!

Directions:

1. Pour your fermented kombucha into a storage container with a lid.

2. Wash strawberries.

3. Add about 10–15 strawberries to your kombucha.

4. Replace the lid and wait 5–7 days to infuse the strawberry flavor.

5. Enjoy!

6. You can either strain the strawberries out and toss them in the compost bin or eat them if you dare!

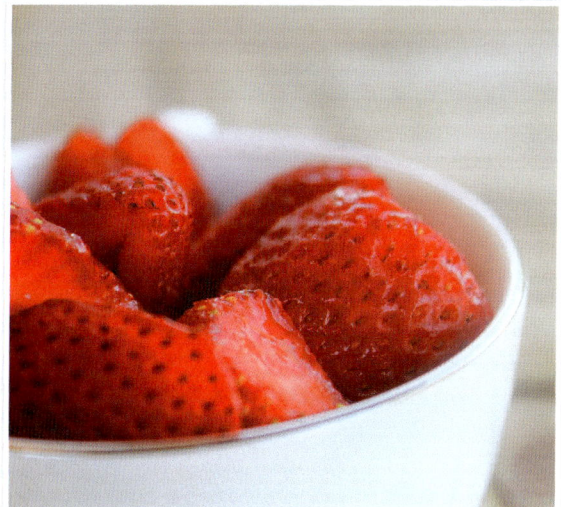

Paleo Made Easy: Getting your Family Started with the Optimal Healthy Lifestyle — with over 45 recipes!

PEACH KOMBUCHA

What you will need:

Kombucha | Peach slices (from 2 peaches) | Air tight storage container | A funnel

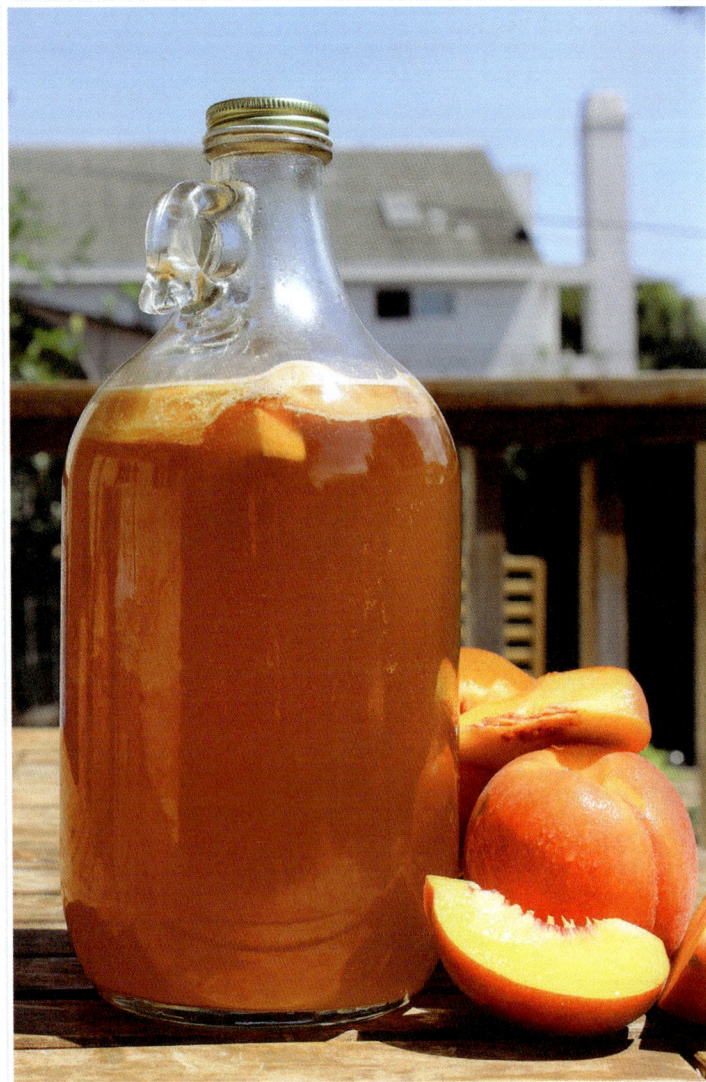

Directions:

1. Pour your kombucha into a storage container with a lid.

2. Wash peaches.

3. Add peach slices to your kombucha.

4. Replace the lid and wait 5–7 days to infuse the peach flavor.

5. Enjoy!

6. You can either strain the peaches out and toss them in the compost bin or eat them if you dare!

Paleo Made Easy: Getting your Family Started with the Optimal Healthy Lifestyle—with over 45 recipes!

HOMEMADE SAUERKRAUT

Fermented foods are a great way to include some good bacteria in your diet!

Similarly to kombucha, sauerkraut is a fermented food that will help keep the flora in your gut well balanced, aiding in digestion and overall health. If you're not up for making your own, you may also be able to find it at your local health food store. Just make sure it's in the refrigerated section (as it should be if it is truly fermented, not filled with a bunch of artificial preservatives) and that the ingredients are cabbage and salt and perhaps a few other recognizable ones for flavor as in the recipe below!

   Making it is super easy and only costs a few cents a batch!

What you will need:

2 medium sized heads of cabbage | 6 tsp. salt | 6 cloves of garlic | 1 tsp. pepper

½ gallon mason jar and cloth to cover (t-shirt material is best) | rubber band

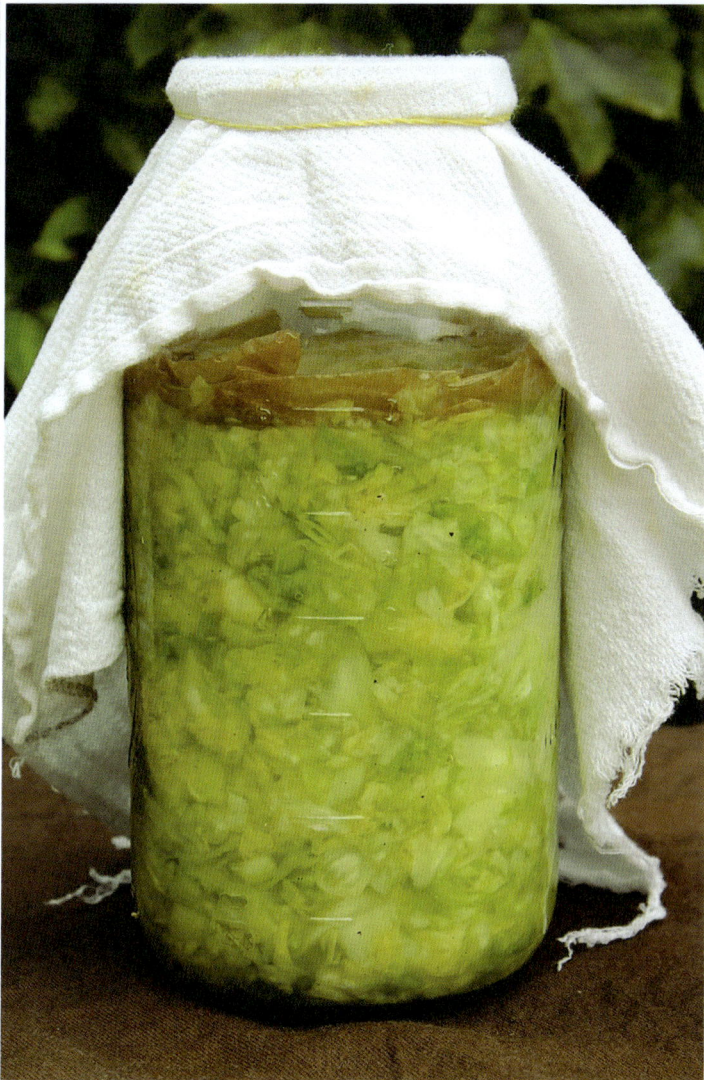

Directions:

1. Chop cabbage (save 1 leaf to cover in jar when finished).

2. Using ⅙ of the cabbage at a time, mix in 1 tsp. salt and mash with hands until liquid begins to emerge. Might take a little elbow grease!

3. Continue this until all cabbage and salt is used.

4. Add garlic and pepper and continue to mix and mash.

5. Once finished fill a ½ gallon mason jar with the cabbage. Liquid should be covering all cabbage.

6. Place the leftover cabbage leaf over the top of the shredded cabbage. Try to get as much air out as possible.

7. Cover jar with a cloth and rubber band and wait 7 days or so. Taste periodically using a clean utensil each time. If a little mold develops simply remove it—it will not affect the rest of it.

8. Once it is to your liking, store with a lid in the refrigerator. It will keep for weeks as the refrigeration will slow down the fermentation quite a bit.

9. Enjoy!

FERMENTED CARROTS

You can ferment just about any vegetable!
All you need is a mason jar, really, but if you want to get fancy you can also use a fermentation crock.

Ingredients

8-10 medium carrots, shredded | 2 cloves of garlic, chopped | 2 Tbsp. sea salt

1 leaf (cabbage preferred but lettuce will work)

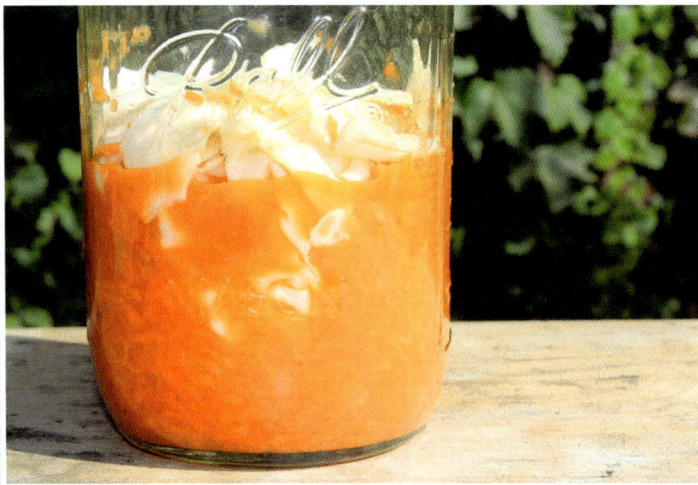

Instructions

1. Shred carrots and place in mixing bowl.

2. Add chopped garlic cloves and sea salt.

3. With your hand, mix the ingredients while squeezing the carrots (the idea is to get the "juice" of the carrots flowing so your mixture will be a quite watery)

4. Patience, keep mixing and squeezing.

5. Place in your glass jar leaving about an inch on the top since it might spill over as it ferments

6. Cover with your cabbage leaf, trying to tuck it in so the carrots are not exposed to air

7. *Optional:* add a weight to hold the cabbage leaf and liquid down. I used a baby food jar filled with water which fit my jar nicely.

8. Recommended: place in a shallow bowl in case spillover (normal!) happens when fermenting

9. Let it sit for 2 weeks checking every other day to make sure its still below water. You can add some filtered water if it gets too dry. Also remove any mold that forms due to air exposure with a clean spoon.

10. When it is done (gauged by taste), place a lid on it and refrigerate.

11. The refrigeration will slow down the fermentation process so it will keep for several weeks.

12. Enjoy!

Paleo Made Easy: Getting your Family Started with the Optimal Healthy Lifestyle—with over 45 recipes!

DIY BASICS AND STAPLES

HOW TO MAKE GELATIN-RICH BONE BROTH

What you will need:

Leftover bones from any pastured animal (I love to add chicken heads and feet since they are especially rich in gelatin)

Filtered water | Slow cooker, pressure cooker, or just a plain old stock pot

1 Tbsp. organic unfiltered apple cider vinegar

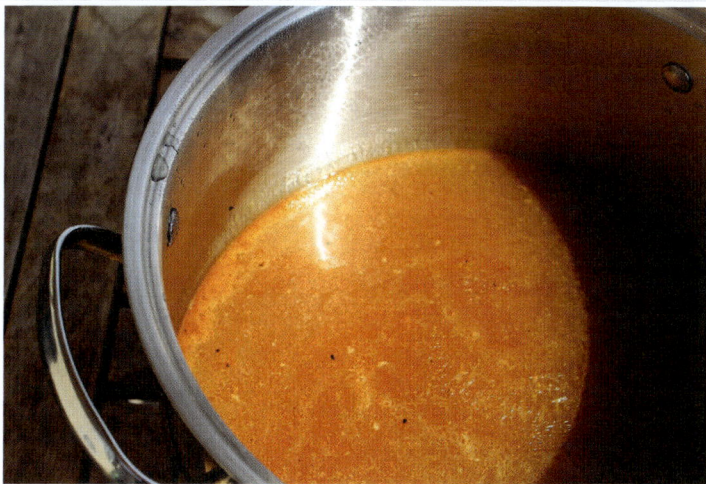

Directions:

1. The slow cooker takes a while to warm up, so we put it on high and add already boiling water. This cuts down on the warm up time. You can also use a pressure cooker or just a pot on the stove but I love the ease of setting the slow cooker on and forgetting it.

2. Add your bones and let cook! Add 1 Tbsp. vinegar (optional). The vinegar helps extract the minerals from the bones, but I find it also makes the broth slightly less palatable. It might take some getting used to, perhaps using just a tiny amount the first few times you do this. We find that if the broth is used to make soup, no one notices. But, when chugging a mug of bone broth, the vinegar flavor is noticeable.

3. Keep adding water if it boils down too far. We usually leave it at least 48 hours.

4. Once you're ready to harvest your broth, pour it through a strainer into a pot and allow it to cool.

5. Use it or freeze it for later!

6. If you want to put the bones in for another round, by all means do it again. Sometimes we get 3 or 4 pots worth of broth from one set of bones!

7. When it cools it may have a thick layer of fat at the top. You can certainly eat it but for some it is tough to digest, so I suggest skimming it off and cooking with it instead.

8. If your broth looks like jello after it has cooled, all the better!

Paleo Made Easy: Getting your Family Started with the Optimal Healthy Lifestyle—with over 45 recipes!

HOMEMADE GRASS-FED GHEE

What is ghee?

Ghee is clarified butter that has been cooked down to separate out the milk proteins (casein),
which some people, like my oldest daughter, are very sensitive to. It is widely used in Indian cooking
and can be used as a replacement for butter or other cooking fats. If you're intolerant to butter and other dairy,
ghee can be a godsend. To me it tastes like candy!

Ingredients:

2 lbs. grass fed butter

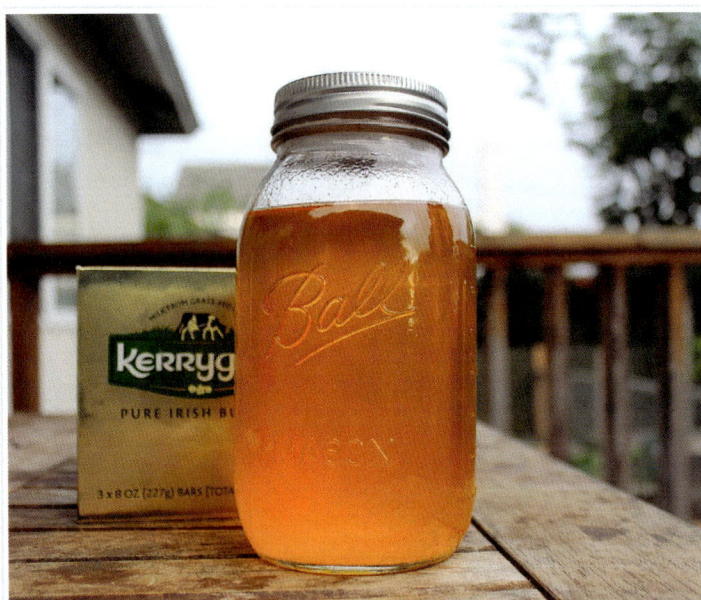

Directions:

1. Place in a pot on LOW heat.

2. Let simmer slowly until it starts to separate, this may take a couple of hours. The lower the heat the better the results—trust me!

3. Curds will first float to top, then sink to bottom.

4. Once it has sunk to the bottom you are ready to filter the Ghee.

5. Pour through some cheese cloth and into a storage container.

6. Let cool.

7. Enjoy!

8. You can store at room temperature or in the fridge—it is up to you!

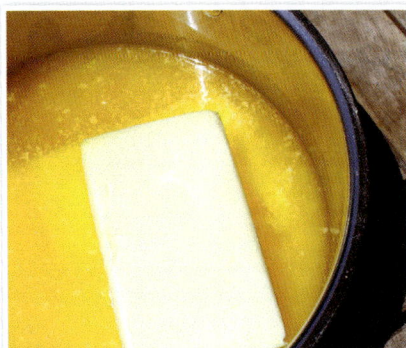
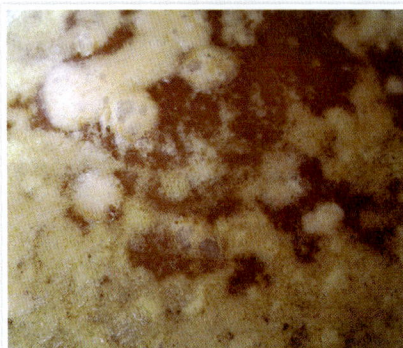
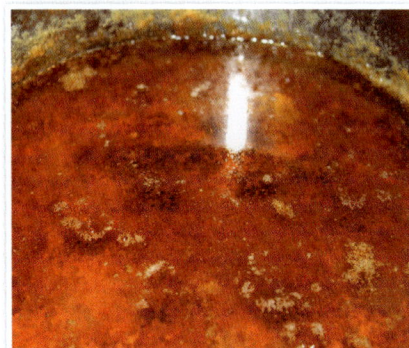

*Paleo Made Easy: Getting your Family Started
with the Optimal Healthy Lifestyle—with over 45 recipes!*

HOMEMADE COCONUT MILK

Coconut milk can be tough to find with no added emulsifiers, preservatives or sweeteners.
And when you do find it, it is expensive and I don't love the waste of all those cans either. I'll be honest,
I buy coconut milk much more often than I make it these days but if you're trying to keep costs down
and ensure the freshness of your milk here is an easy recipe!

What you will need:

2 cups of shredded coconut | 3 cups of boiling filtered water | A nut milk bag

A food processor or blender

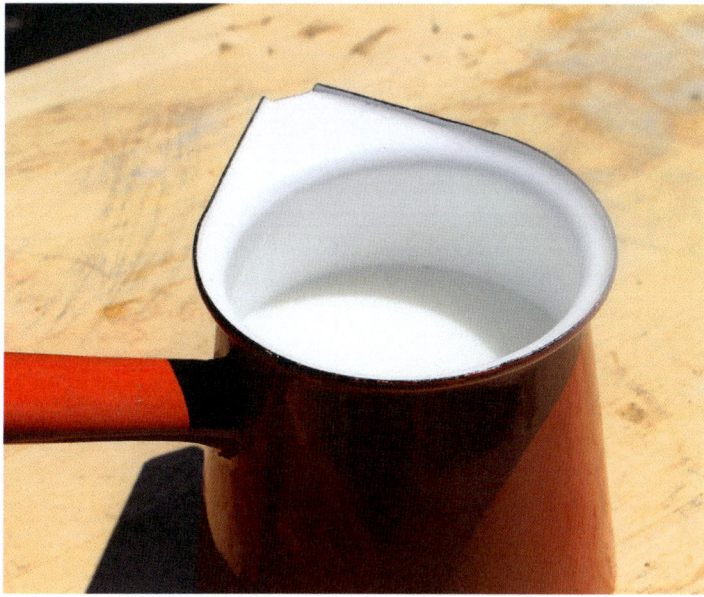

Directions:

1. Put the shredded coconut and the boiling water in the processor.

2. Blend it well for 2 minutes!

3. After letting it cool pour it through your strainer into a small bowl.

4. Squeeze as much milk as you can from the remaining coconut.

5. Enjoy!

*Paleo Made Easy: Getting your Family Started
with the Optimal Healthy Lifestyle—with over 45 recipes!*

CONDIMENTS AND SAUCES

CREAMY TURMERIC SAUCE (ANTI-INFLAMMATORY, AIP FRIENDLY)

Turmeric, which is native to India and part of the ginger family, has long been used in medicine. It is a powerful anti-inflammatory. It also has a lot of other great benefits, like reducing insulin levels, fighting cancer, and speeding up healing[20].

Please note: Turmeric does stain clothing if very concentrated, so use carefully!
Sauces are a great way to get turmeric into your diet while adding a little spice to your food!
This recipe has become a staple in our house.

Ingredients:

3 cans (13.5oz) coconut milk | 2 teaspoons salt | 1 tsp turmeric | 1 tsp garlic powder | 1 tsp onion powder

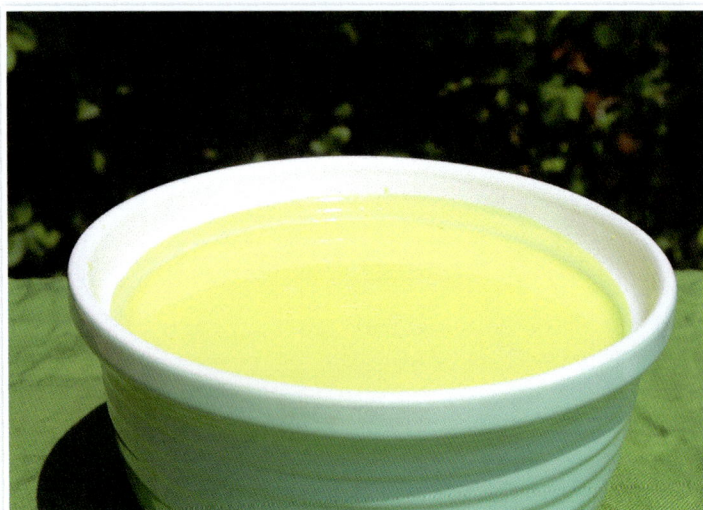

Instructions:

1. Pour coconut milk into a saucepan (12" works well).

2. Add all the spices.

3. Mix well and bring to a boil.

4. Let simmer to thicken the sauce for 15–30 minutes—the longer it simmers, the stronger the flavor and the thicker the sauce.

The kids LOVE this stuff. They want it slathered on their burgers and vegetables and like to use it as dipping sauce. Enjoy!

Paleo Made Easy: Getting your Family Started with the Optional Healthy Lifestyle—with over 45 recipes!

HOMEMADE PALEO BACONNAISE

It's no secret that we love our bacon. We also love bacon fat! Store bought mayo often contains rancid seed oils and other questionable ingredients. If you have a few minutes, it's best to make your own.

What you will need:

Food processor or a whisk and some stamina | ½ cup olive oil | ½ cup bacon fat, preferably pastured

2 large egg yolks | 1 Tbsp. lemon juice | 2 tsp. apple cider vinegar

½ tsp. gluten-free mustard | ½ tsp. salt

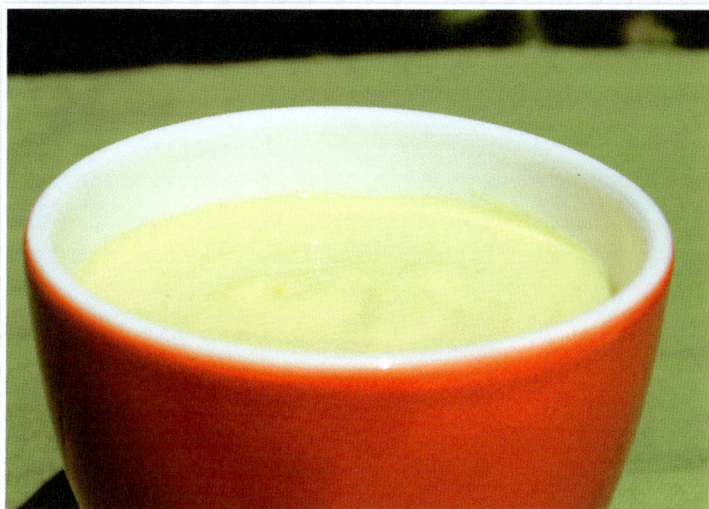

Directions:

1. Combine the egg yolk, lemon juice, vinegar, mustard and salt in a food processor or bowl.

2. Mix until blended and bright yellow.

3. Use the drip function on the food processor to slowly add the olive oil while the processor is mixing or add ¼ tsp. at a time while whisking by hand.

4. Slowly add the bacon fat (you may have to warm it in order to pour it in) in the same way as the olive oil.

5. Mix until you get the consistency you want—it will not be as firm as store-bought mayo, but it will be spreadable once it spends some time in the fridge.

6. Enjoy!

Paleo Made Easy: Getting your Family Started with the Optimal Healthy Lifestyle—with over 45 recipes!

CREAMY TOMATO ROSEMARY SAUCE

Ingredients:

3 medium size tomatoes | ¼ cup ghee | 1 white onion | Cream from 3 cans of coconut milk

1.5 tsp. sea salt | ½ tsp. pepper | Leaves from 2 sprigs of fresh rosemary

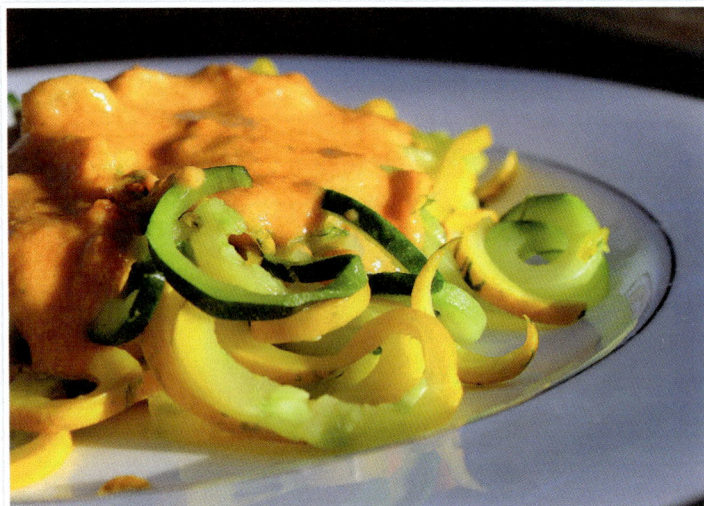

Directions:

1. Put ghee in a saucepan on medium heat.

2. Add rosemary and chopped onion.

3. Cook until onion is translucent.

4. Add chopped tomatoes, coconut milk cream, salt and pepper.

5. Stir ingredients until they soften.

6. Remove from heat and pour into blender or food processor.

7. Process until smooth.

8. Pour back into saucepan and reduce until desired thickness.

9. Enjoy!

Serve over zucchini noodles which are easily made with a spiral vegetable slicer and cooking the zucchini noodles lightly in a saucepan.

SIMPLE SALSA

What you will need:

6 tomatoes, chopped | 3 large cloves of fresh garlic, minced | 1 green bell pepper, chopped

1 small red onion, chopped | 2 Tbsp. EVOO | Juice from one lime | ¼ cup fresh parsley, chopped

Chili powder, salt, and pepper to taste

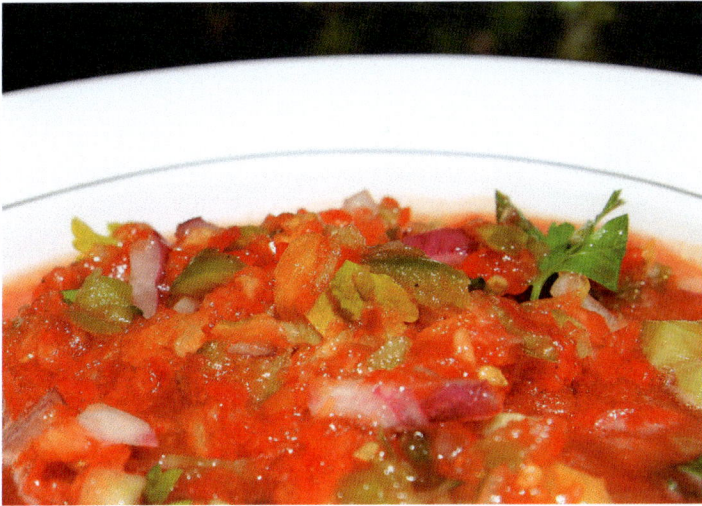

Directions:

1. Place tomatoes in the food processor and blend until chunky and pour into a bowl.

2. Repeat step 1 with the onions, bell pepper and parsley.

3. Combine all ingredients in the bowl and mix well.

4. Enjoy!

BACON GUACAMOLE

Some days we get lazy and just mash some avocado in a bowl and call it guacamole :)

Other days we get crazy and start tossing stuff in it, like bacon fat!
Why not (it's pastured bacon, of course!) This recipe is delicious!

What you will need:

5–7 large avocados | ⅛ cup bacon fat | 3 cloves of garlic | 1 medium tomato | ½ lemon

1 small red onion | 1 tsp. sea salt | dash of cayenne pepper

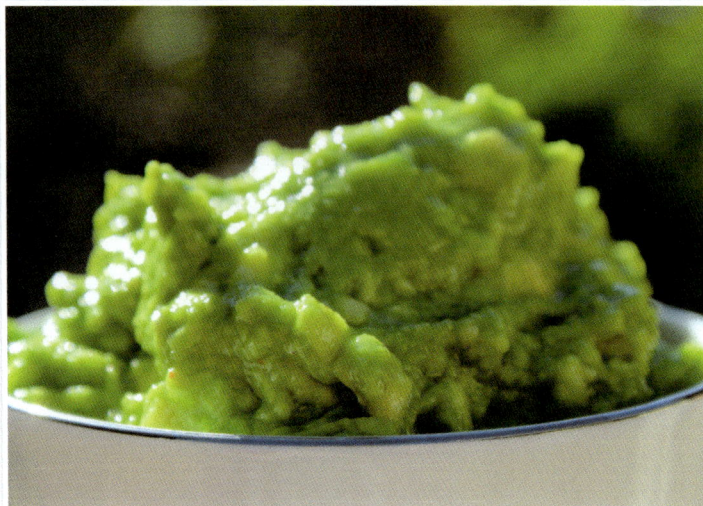

Directions:

1. Cut avocados into small chunks and place in a large bowl.

2. Mince garlic and add.

3. Chop tomato and onion finely and add.

4. Add juice from ½ lemon.

5. Heat bacon fat in a small pan until it is liquid and add.

6. Add 1 tsp. sea salt.

7. Mash mixture and mix well.

8. Enjoy! We love to dip sliced jicama in it!

Paleo Made Easy: Getting your Family Started with the Optimal Healthy Lifestyle—with over 45 recipes!

PALEO CHICKEN CURRY

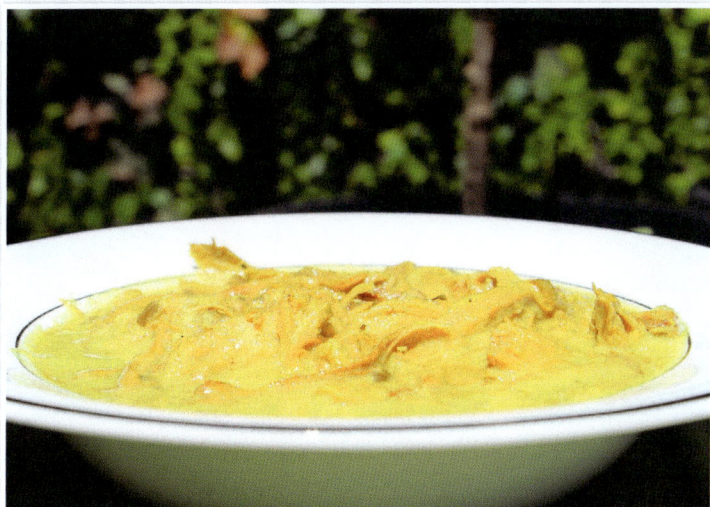

Instructions

1. Place chopped onion in a skillet with the ghee and rosemary.

2. Cook until translucent.

3. Add the remainder of the ingredients and mix well.

4. Let simmer until the desired consistency—the longer the more flavorful!

5. Enjoy over cauliflower rice!

CHIMICHURRI

Ingredients:

½ cup Olive Oil | ½ cup (approx) of chopped fresh parsley | 4 garlic cloves | ½ Tbsp salt

½ tsp of pepper | the juice of half a lemon | 4–6 leaves of chopped fresh basil (optional)

⅛ tsp cayenne (optional)

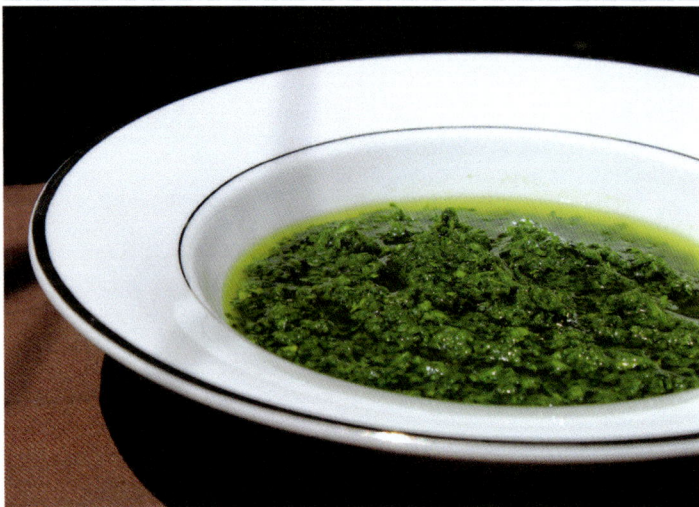

Directions:

1. Blend all ingredients except the olive oil in a food processor

2. Once ingredients are processed put them in a separate bowl

3. Add the olive oil and mix with a spoon

4. Enjoy!

DESSERTS

KOMBUCHA POPSICLES

I checked with my friend and fermenting expert Hannah Crum from Kombuchakamp.com for her thoughts on whether freezing kombucha would kill ALL the probiotic benefits of it.

She said:

"Even if the probiotics die, and it's hard to say if they would revive in the stomach, the beneficial acids/vitamins & other stuff are all still there. There's also research that dead bacteria can pass DNA signatures onto living bacteria enabling them to still have a positive influence. All in all, it's good to get more booch in the diet however you like to do it".

Works for me!

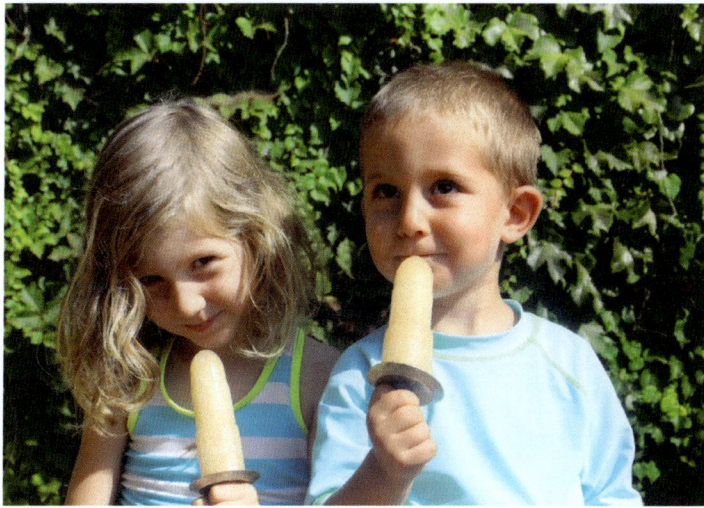

How To Make Kombucha Popsicles

1. Brew kombucha (instructions on page 59)
2. Pour "booch" in molds
3. Freeze
4. Serve!

I'm serious, that's all I did. They love it!

Paleo Made Easy: Getting your Family Started with the Optimal Healthy Lifestyle—with over 45 recipes!

SNEAKY GREEN POPSICLES!

So, my kids will eat chicken feet but they push spinach around on their plates...

The only greens they're into at the moment are kale chips. The reason for choosing spinach for these popsicles is that it is high in magnesium, which is great for the growing pains my 4 year old has been having. (I also put epsom salts in her bath each night which has helped quite a bit!). Inspired by the kombucha popsicles, which were such a hit and hardly sweet at all, I figured I'd test the limits to what they'll *eat as long as it is frozen.*

Disclaimer: I'm not huge on the idea of sneaking foods to your kids without them knowing. In fact, in this book, you'll only see it done twice: these popsicles and the liver burgers on page 45. I much prefer teaching kids about what foods are nourishing and having their palate adapt over time. But hey, sometimes you just gotta do what you gotta do.

Ingredients

2 (13.5 oz) cans of coconut milk | 1 bag frozen chopped spinach | 2 tablespoons vanilla

1 tablespoon maple syrup (optional)

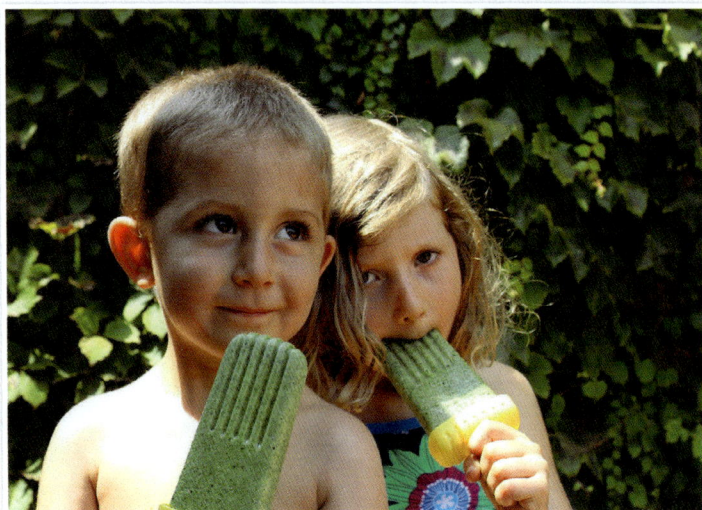

Instructions

1. Put everything in the food processor or blender and blend the heck out of it.

2. The more blended, the better.

3. Pour into the popsicle molds and freeze (at least 4 hours)

4. Enjoy!

Verdict? Adult and kid approved!

Paleo Made Easy: Getting your Family Started with the Optimal Healthy Lifestyle—with over 45 recipes!

FRENCH VANILLA CHOCOLATE CHIP ICE CREAM

Ice cream is one of the things we don't eat very often because it's hard to find good coconut milk ice cream at the store which doesn't have carrageenan or highly processed sweeteners like agave and aspartame. So we bought an ice cream maker so we can do it ourselves. Problem solved!

What you will need:

An ice cream maker | 2 eggs, preferably pastured | 1 Tbsp. vanilla | 2 cans Organic Coconut Milk

½ cup organic grade "B" maple syrup | ¼ cup dairy free, soy free chocolate chips

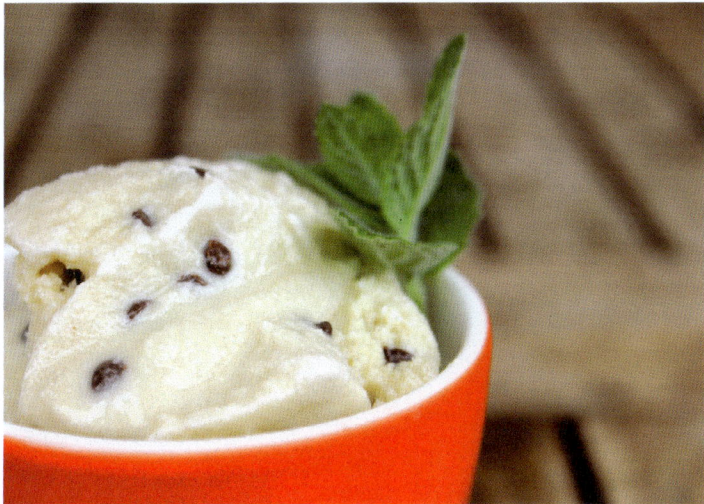

Directions:

1. Mix the coconut milk, eggs, vanilla and maple syrup in a bowl or blender for approximately 2 minutes or until blended well.

2. Pour the contents into your ice cream maker and turn on for 20 minutes.

3. Add the chocolate chips and let run for another 10 minutes.

4. Turn off and empty contents into an airtight container and place in the freezer for approximately 3 hours.

5. Take out and enjoy!

BANANA TARTS (21-DAY SUGAR DETOX APPROVED!)

If you've been following my blog or Facebook page, you'll know I do a 21 Day Sugar Detox a couple times a year if I feel like the desserts have been making too frequent an appearance and I just want to "reset". This program is as close as I come to a diet these days. One of my best tricks for success is to have a treat available which won't derail the success of the detox. These Banana Tarts are perfect for that! If you're not on the detox, I would add a bit of raw honey or maple syrup because they're definitely mild. If you are on the detox, these might be a lifesaver! For more info on the detox program please visit: www. hollywoodhomestead.com/21DSD

What you will need:

½ cup coconut cream concentrate

1 large or 2 small green tipped bananas (if not on the detox, regular bananas will work) | 3 Tbsp. coconut oil

1 Tbsp. vanilla | 1 tsp. cinnamon | A pinch of salt | Silicone muffin pan

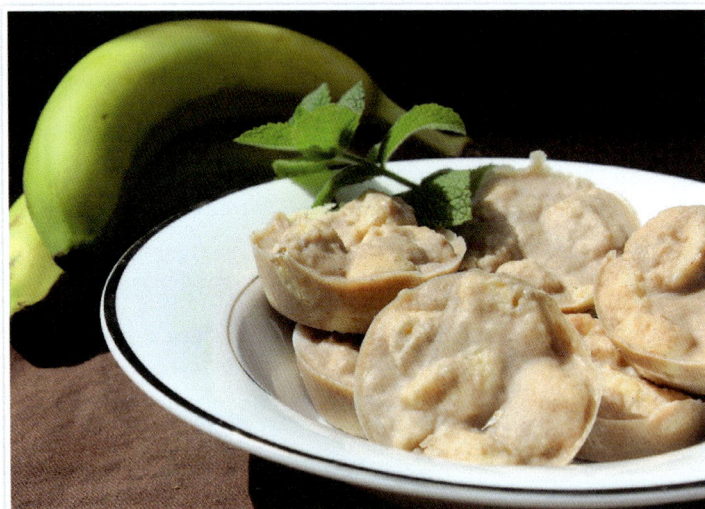

Directions:

1. Mix all ingredients except banana well. You may need to warm the coconut cream concentrate in the microwave or on the stovetop in order to mix it.

2. Cut bananas into small square chunks and add to the mixture.

3. Use a small amount of coconut oil to grease the muffin pan (approx. 9 spots).

4. Pour mixture in to the muffin pan.

5. Place in fridge for 15 minutes.

6. Enjoy!

Paleo Made Easy: Getting your Family Started with the Optimal Healthy Lifestyle—with over 45 recipes!

CHOCOLATE DIPPED STRAWBERRIES

What you will need:

3 pints of strawberries | ½ cup of dairy free, soy free chocolate chips

The cream from 2 cans of coconut milk (the cream separates from the milk as long as you don't shake it up!)

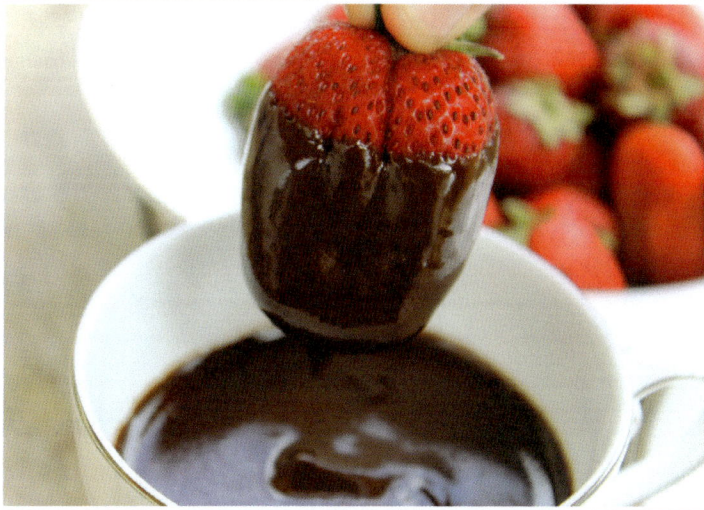

Directions:

1. Skim the cream from the 2 cans of coconut milk and spoon into a saucepan on low heat.

2. Add the chocolate chips and stir well until melted and smooth.

3. Pour the chocolate into a container for dipping.

4. Dip the strawberries into the chocolate. Either eat on the spot or place in the fridge until the chocolate hardens.

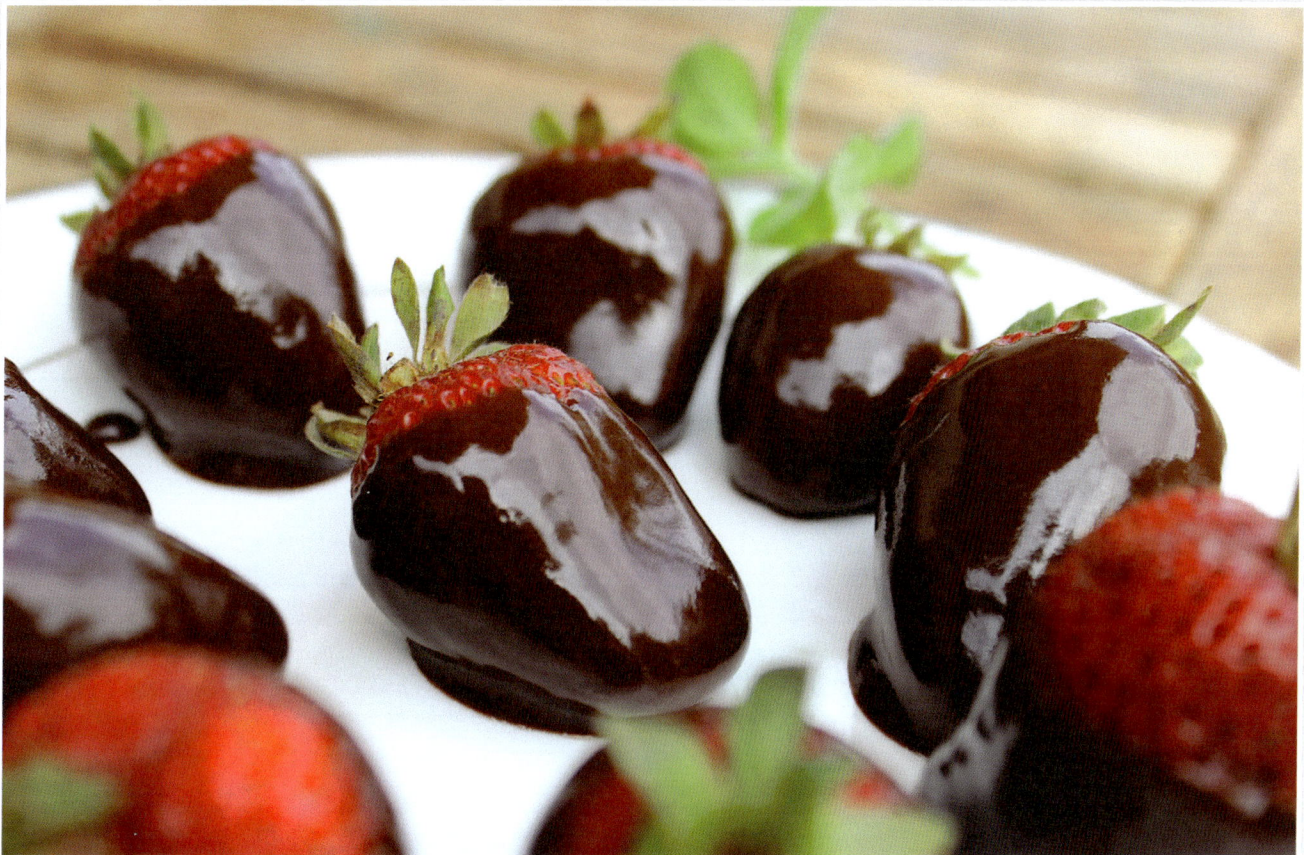

5. Enjoy!

Paleo Made Easy: Getting your Family Started with the Optimal Healthy Lifestyle — with over 45 recipes!

MOJITO SORBET

For a great summer treat, how about a refreshing recipe for a mojito sorbet!
With or without rum, it is delicious!

What you will need:

Ice cream maker | 1 cup water | 1 cup sparkling water | ¾ cup maple syrup | ¼ cup mint leaves, packed | ⅛ cup grated lime zest | ¾ cup fresh lime juice | 2 Tbsp. rum (optional)

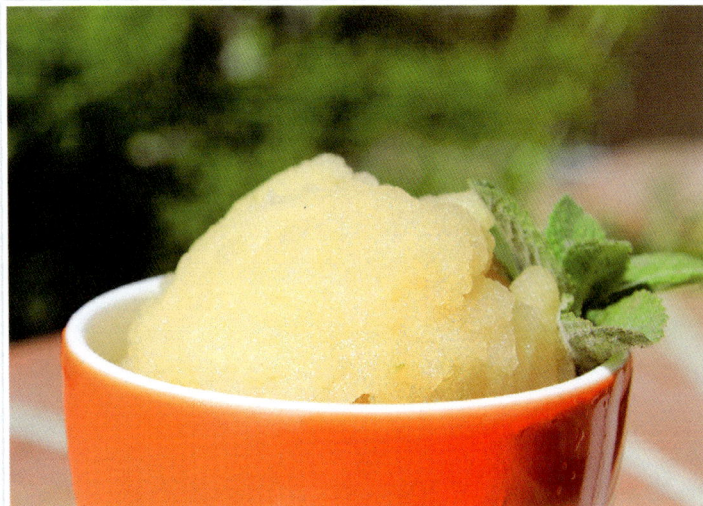

Directions:

1. Heat the water, maple syrup, mint leaves and zest in a saucepan over medium heat.

2. Bring to a boil, reduce heat, and simmer for 5 minutes.

3. Strain out the mint leaves and zest and set aside to cool.

4. Once cool, add lime juice, water and optional rum into the bowl and mix well.

5. Pour into ice cream maker and allow to mix for 30 minutes.

6. Enjoy!

WARM CINNAMON APPLESAUCE (SUGAR FREE)

When I first transitioned my kids to a real food diet,
I was surprised to find out just how many of the products I was buying had wonky ingredients in them—
like high fructose corn syrup, loads of unnecessary refined sugar, or unpronounceable chemicals.

I was shocked that even applesauce was one of those products... I guess I fell for the apples on the label. They must have forgotten to include the photo of the high fructose corn syrup. I mean, applesauce should really be just that: apples cooked until soft enough to become sauce consistency.

My kids LOVE applesauce and of course the stuff I was buying was no bueno. Luckily, homemade applesauce is super easy to make ahead and freeze for the kids or for yourself! This recipe is Fall-inspired and is best served warm.

Ingredients

8 organic apples (I like Fuji apples) | 1 cup of filtered water | 1 tsp ground cinnamon | 2 Tbsp. grass-fed ghee

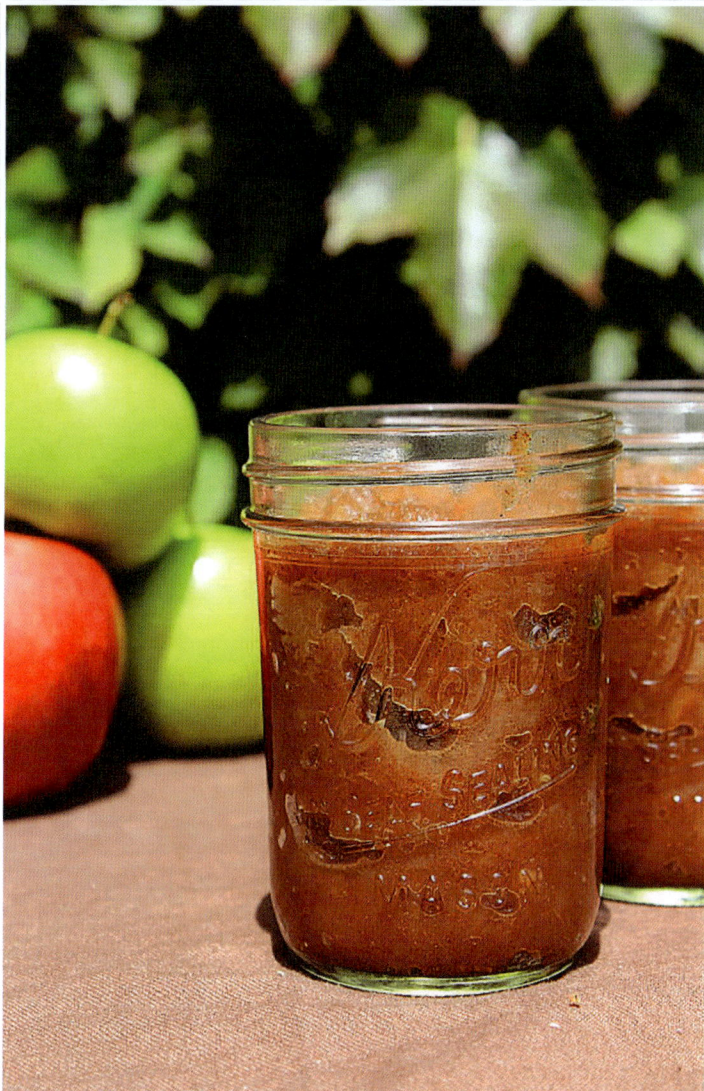

Directions

1. Peel, core and roughly chop apples.

2. Place all ingredients into a pan on medium/high heat.

3. Mix until simmering.

4. Cover and turn down to low/medium heat.

5. After 20–30 minutes take off the stove and mash or put in food processor.

6. Serve warm and enjoy!

*Paleo Made Easy: Getting your Family Started
with the Optimal Healthy Lifestyle—with over 45 recipes!*

BACON WRAPPED DATES STUFFED WITH GUACAMOLE

Ingredients:

20 large dates | 1 pound of bacon | 1 cup of Guacamole | 1 box of toothpicks

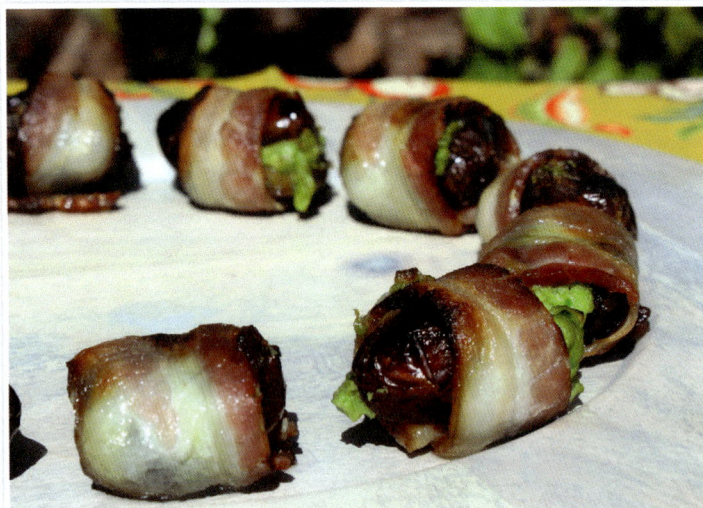

Directions:

1. Place bacon on pans and place in the oven for 15 minutes at 350 degrees

2. While the bacon is cooking remove the pits from the dates and stuff with guacamole

3. Take the bacon out of the oven and cut each piece in half

4. Wrap each stuffed date with ½ piece of bacon and use the toothpicks to secure them

5. Place the finished product on a baking pan and put in the over for 20 minutes at 350 degrees or until bacon is crispy

6. Enjoy!

GELATIN SNACKS

We love sneaking grass-fed gelatin into our diets,
especially when it is too warm to be drinking bone broth. It is just like eating bones!
It doesn't get more paleo than that.

Grass fed gelatin is also great source of collagen, you know the stuff people inject in their lips and foreheads? Its edible botox! :)

HOMEMADE ORANGE JELLO

Have you seen the list of ingredients in store-bought jello? It's like reading a bad novel.
This recipe is simple and healthy!

Ingredients:

2 cups orange juice | 2 T. grass fed gelatin

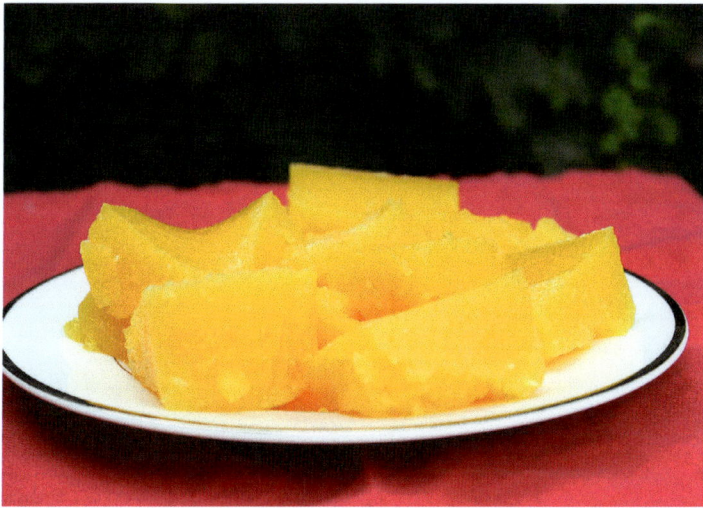

Directions:

1. Pour ½ cup of orange juice into saucepan on low heat.

2. Pour in your gelatin and mix well until dissolved.

3. Pour in the remaining juice and turn off heat.

4. Pour gelatin into a glass bowl.

5. Let cool and place in the fridge for at least 3 hours.

6. Enjoy!

*Paleo Made Easy: Getting your Family Started
with the Optimal Healthy Lifestyle — with over 45 recipes!*

ORANGE GUMMIES

We are lucky enough to have a huge orange tree in our back yard, so we are always looking for new ways to take advantage of the oranges we have.

Ingredients:

⅓ cup of juiced oranges | 3 Tbsp. Grass Fed Gelatin

2–3 Tbsp. Raw Honey (I find that 2 is plenty but some might like it sweeter)

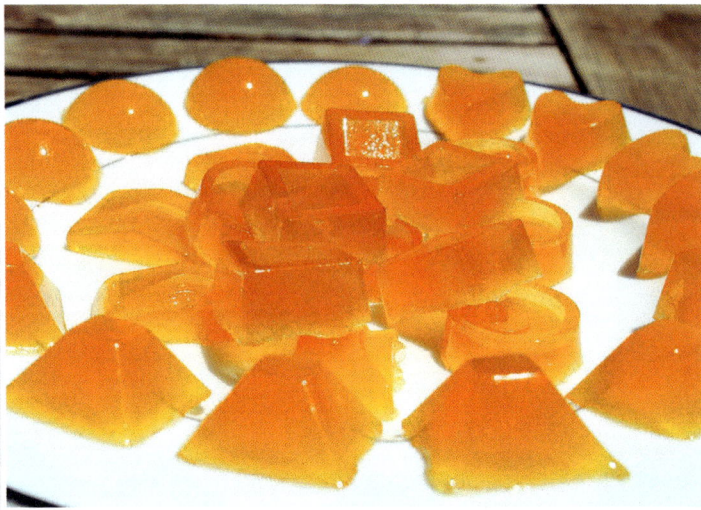

Directions:

1. Put all ingredients in a saucepan. Heat just enough so everything dissolves, stirring constantly. Don't let it come to a boil because you'll kill the awesome probiotic qualities in the raw honey.

2. Pour into silicone molds.

3. Place in the freezer for 10 minutes. I wish I could tell you how long they last but, in my house, things last about 30 seconds unless I hide them!

4. Enjoy!

Paleo Made Easy: Getting your Family Started with the Optimal Healthy Lifestyle—with over 45 recipes!

STRAWBERRY LEMONADE GUMMIES

What you will need:

1 cup pureed strawberries | ⅓ cup lemon juice | 2 Tbsp. raw honey

9 Tbsp. grass-fed gelatin | Silicone molds

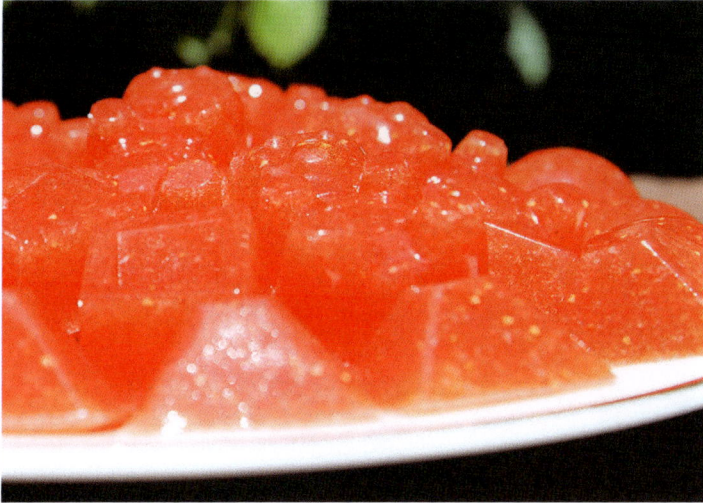

Directions:

1. Put strawberry mixture, lemon juice and honey into a saucepan. Cook on low/medium heat.

2. Mix well until warm (not hot as it will kill the probiotic properties of the raw honey!).

3. Add gelatin and mix well until dissolved.

4. Pour contents of pan into a cup with a spout (like a measuring cup).

5. Pour mixture into candy molds.

6. Place in freezer for 15 minutes.

7. Enjoy!

Paleo Made Easy: Getting your Family Started with the Optimal Healthy Lifestyle—with over 45 recipes!

LEMON GUMMIES

What you will need:

⅓ cup fresh-squeezed lemon juice | 3 Tbsp. grass-fed gelatin | 2 Tbsp. raw honey*

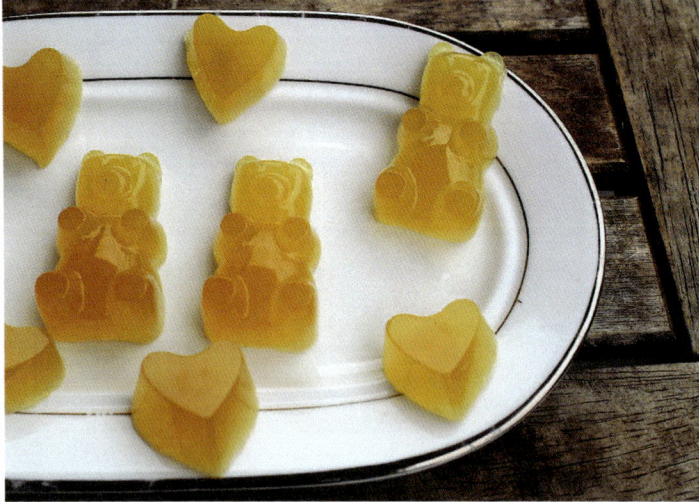

Directions:

1. Put lemon juice and honey into a skillet and cook on low heat- don't let it get too hot since it will kill the probiotic awesomeness of the raw honey!

2. Once warm, mix in the gelatin.

3. Mix thoroughly until the gelatin has dissolved.

4. Pour into a measuring cup, and then into molds

5. Put in freezer for 15 minutes.

6. Take out and enjoy!

*If you or your kids are used to sweeter foods you may want to start with more and as time goes by you can experiment with reducing the quantity.

REFERENCES

1. Gunnars, Kris. "Grass-Fed vs Grain-Fed Beef—What's The Difference?" *Authority Nutrition*, 8 Aug 2013. Web. 5 Oct 2013. authoritynutrition.com

2. Ballantyne, Sarah, Ph.D. "Grass-Fed Beef: A Superfood worth the Premium Price." *The Paleo Mom*, 20 March 2012. Web. 5 Oct 2013. www.thepaleomom.com

3. "Grass fed meat: what's all the hype?" *Paleoscape*, 3 March 2011. Web. 5 Oct 2013. www.paleoscape.com

4. Enig, Mary G., Ph.D. "Importance of Saturated Fats for Biological Functions." *Weston A. Price Foundation*, 8 July 2004. Web. 5 Oct 2013. www.westonaprice.org

5. Knopp, Robert H. and Barbara M. Retzlaff. "Saturated fat prevents coronary artery disease? An American paradox." *American Journal of Clinical Nutrition* 80.5 (2004): 1102-1103.

6. Hoenselaar, Robert. "Saturated fat and cardiovascular disease: The discrepancy between the scientific literature and dietary advice." *Nutrition* 28 (2012): 118-123.

7. Kresser, Chris. "New study puts final nail in the 'saturated fat causes heart disease' coffin." ChrisKresser.com. 15 Jan 2010. Web. 5 Oct 2013. chriskresser.com

8. "EWG's Shopper's Guide to Pesticides in Produce 2013." *Environmental Working Group*. Web. 5 Oct 2013. www.ewg.org

9. Nagel, Ramiel. "Living with Phytic Acid." *Weston A. Price Foundation*, 5 March 2010. Web. 5 Oct 2013. www.westonaprice.org

10. Kresser, Chris. "Liver: nature's most potent superfood." *Chris Kresser*. 11 April 2008. Web. 5 Oct 2013. chriskresser.com

11. Ballantyne, Sarah, Ph.D. "Why Everyone Should Be Eating Organ Meat." *The Paleo Mom*, 7 April 2012. Web. 5 Oct 2013. www.thepaleomom.com

12. *Nutrition Data.* nutritiondata.self.com

13. Crow, Catherine. "Gelatin and Collagen Hydrolysate—What's the Difference?" *The Healthy Home Economist*, 19 Aug 2013. Web. 5 Oct 2013. www.thehealthyhomeeconomist.com

14. Micleu, Cindy, MTCM, LAc. "Bone Broth for Building: Nourishing the Liver and Kidneys." *Jade Institute*. Web. 5 Oct 2013. www.jadeinstitute.com

15. "Gelatin: Do You know this Superfood?" *Savory Lotus*, 22 May 2013. Web. 5 Oct 2013. http://www.savorylotus.com

16. Ballantyne, Sarah, Ph.D. "Teaser Excerpt from The Paleo Approach—The Importance of Sleep." *The Paleo Mom*, 4 April 2012. Web. 5 Oct 2013. www.thepaleomom.com

17. Kresser, Chris. "How Artificial Light is Wrecking Your Sleep and What to Do About It." ChrisKresser.com. 22 Feb 2013. Web. 5 Oct 2013. chriskresser.com

18. Sisson, Mark. "How Light Affects Our Sleep." *Mark's Daily Apple*, 4 March 2010. Web. 5 Oct 2013. www.marksdailyapple.com

19. Graves, Ginny. "How Exercise Can Make You Happy." *Self*, May 2012. Web. 5 Oct 2013. www.self.com.

20. Sisson, Mark. "Smart Spice: Turmeric." *Mark's Daily Apple*, 25 May 2010. Web. 5 Oct 2013. www.marksdailyapple.com

Printed in Great Britain
by Amazon